Child Protection: A Guide for Midwives

2nd edition

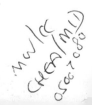

For *Books for Midwives:*

Commissioning Editor: *Mary Seager*
Development Editor: *Catharine Steers*
Project Manager: *Ailsa Laing*
Designer: *George Ajayi*

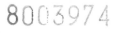

Child Protection: A Guide for Midwives

2nd edition

Jenny Fraser MSc RM RN DPSM
Norfolk & Norwich University Hospital NHS Trust, Norwich, UK

with

Mary Nolan PhD MA BA(Hons) RGN
Antenatal Teacher/Tutor, The National Childbirth Trust, UK

FOREWORD BY

Paul Howard
Head of Norfolk Constabulary Child Protection Team 1995–2002

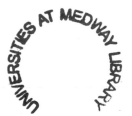

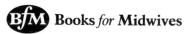 **Books** *for* **Midwives**

Edinburgh London New York Oxford Philadelphia St Louis Sydney Toronto 2004

Books for Midwives
An imprint of Elsevier Limited

First edition 1997
Second edition 2004

ISBN 0 7506 5352 3

British Library Cataloguing in Publication Data
A catalogue record for this book is available from the British Library

Library of Congress Cataloging in Publication Data
A catalog record for this book is available from the Library of
Congress

Medical knowledge is constantly changing. Standard safety
precautions must be followed, but as new research and clinical
experience broaden our knowledge, changes in treatment and drug
therapy may become necessary or appropriate. Readers are advised
to check the most current product information provided by the
manufacturer of each drug to be administered to verify the
recommended dose, the method and duration of administration,
and contraindications. It is the responsibility of the practitioner,
relying on experience and knowledge of the patient, to determine
dosages and the best treatment for each individual patient. Neither
the Publisher nor the author assumes any liability for any injury
and/or damage to persons or property arising from this publication.

The Publisher

Printed in China

The
Publisher's
policy is to use
**paper manufactured
from sustainable forests**

Contents

Abbreviations used within this book

ACPC	area child protection committee
CAFCASS	Children and Family Court Advisory and Support Services
CPC	child protection committee
DH	Department of Health
EPO	emergency protection order
FCWS	Family Court Welfare Services
GALRO	Guardian *Ad Litem* and Reporting Officer Service
GP	general practitioner
ICO	interim care order
NICU	neonatal intensive care unit
NMC	Nursing and Midwifery Council
NSPCC	National Society for the Prevention of Cruelty to Children
PTSD	post-traumatic stress disorder
SCR	serious case review

Foreword

Safeguarding children from harm is the responsibility of everybody in this country. This means not only professionals from the statutory, voluntary and independent sectors, but also the general public.

However, particular professionals are charged with a special responsibility to ensure that children are protected. These include, among others, the social services, the police, the many facets of the health services, the probation and education services and the NSPCC.

It is a little known fact that there are more police officers in this country working solely on child protection than there are in the national crime squad, who are tasked with targeting the top flight criminal fraternity. This tells something of the importance that the police service places on child protection work.

Officers on child protection units undergo specialist training, they are continually kept up-to-date and their performance is monitored. Proposals are in hand to have a national curriculum of training, together with a requirement that officers must possess certain core competencies before they can undertake child protection work. Having said that, child protection issues are the responsibility of every officer and civilian in the police services, a fact they are continually reminded of.

The same responsibility applies to all professionals, and midwives are no exception. It is the duty of health services to provide adequate training for their entire staff; the level of which would depend on their particular roles and responsibility. However, staff should also update and educate themselves in this complex area of work.

The second edition of this book about child protection is an excellent guide for midwives, who should all make sure that they have a copy, because it clearly sets out their role in child protection, and also provides the fuller picture. It helps midwives to understand the role of the other agencies and the powers available to them. In a time of greater accountability, it is essential that everyone not only understands their responsibility, but also where they fit into the greater scheme of things. This book contributes greatly to that knowledge.

Sadly it may never be possible to fully eradicate child abuse, but better knowledge and more professional working practices will most certainly bring about a reduction.

Paul Howard
Retired Detective Inspector with the Norfolk Constabulary
Head of Norfolk Constabulary Child Protection Team
1995–2002

Preface

Child protection has become more and more a part of most midwives' working lives. It is a subject that midwives usually find upsetting and unsettling, as the thrust of midwifery care is to enable and empower mothers and fathers to become loving and capable parents. It can therefore be difficult for midwives when they become caught up with parents who are involved with child protection processes.

Dealing with parents who may not be allowed to take their babies home with them demands a different approach from the midwife, with which she may not always feel comfortable. Through their years in practice, midwives will become a little used to sending parents home without their baby following a stillbirth, but dealing with parents whose baby is going to someone else's home is even more difficult. In addition, for the parents it is a time of intense scrutiny from different professional agencies, while in hospital and again once home in the community. This can cause a great deal of anger and upset and the midwife may be caught up in a fraught situation. There is also the possibility that a court order needs to be secured to keep the baby safe, and sometimes this may involve the midwife in a court attendance.

The midwife may find herself caring for a woman who has no means of support. She may have a partner who is abusive and violent towards her; she may want him to be at the birth but his behaviour is such that he is ejected from the birth because of a fear of violence towards the woman or staff. The woman may not know who made her pregnant; she may know but choose not to tell for fear of recrimination – it may be her pimp or a relative. She may be a chaotic drug user, she may be homeless, she may be a prostitute. Midwives need to be mindful and considerate to women caught up in child protection procedures and have due regard to the difficulties of their situation. Midwives need to consider that if these particular women had enjoyed a happy and fruitful life with their own parents then, in all probability, they would not be enduring the rigours of the child protection process.

There are many successful projects up and down the country which target such vulnerable women, and prevent some of these women becoming involved with child protection procedures. There are many examples of such practices published regularly in the midwifery journals and it is well worth taking note of such articles and publications. The midwife can learn a great deal by familiarizing herself with alternative ways of working, and by thinking about whether a scheme to target and support vulnerable women could be undertaken in her own area.

This book has been written specifically for midwives and should deepen a midwife's knowledge of the subject as it attempts to demystify some of the practices necessary within child protection. It can be used as an ongoing reference tool and dipped into time and again as you gain more confidence and understanding of the process. For this reason, some things are repeated in different chapters – in case the midwife consults only one chapter when in search of information. The female pronoun has been used for midwives and social workers to avoid being cumbersome and is not in any way intended to be sexist. To differentiate, any child is referred to by the masculine pronoun.

Any child protection work requires professionals from different disciplines and agencies to work together. Multidisciplinary working among health workers will involve midwives working with health visitors, nurses, hospital doctors and GPs. Multiagency working is between the aforementioned health workers and other agencies, namely social services and the police. Health, social services and the police are the three main strands involved in child protection procedures. Other agencies that may become involved are the probation services, legal services (i.e. solicitors) and education.

Child protection is governed by statute and the relevant laws are the 'Children Act 1989' for England and Wales and the 'Children (Scotland) Act 1995' for children living in Scotland. The implementation of these Acts involved radical changes to childcare law and these are discussed in detail in Chapter 8. The book will deal with the implications of these changes with a particular focus on their relevance to midwives.

There are two vital publications which are referred to throughout this book. The first is a publication which was prepared jointly by the Department of Health, the Home Office and the Department for Education and Employment and is called *Working Together to Safeguard Children: A guide to inter-agency working to safeguard and promote the welfare of children* (1999). The equivalent publication for Scotland, prepared by the Scottish Office, is called *Protecting Children – A Shared Responsibility: Guidance on Inter-agency Co-operation* (1998). The Stationery Office (TSO) publishes both publications, and a full list of bookshops is provided in the Appendix.

These publications require local authorities to set out good practice in order to implement the provisions of the two Acts. Neither of the publications, *Working Together* or *Protecting Children*, has the full force of statute, but their recommendations for practice are expected to be complied with. The publications have enabled uniformity of actions regarding child protection throughout the different agencies involved, which should streamline the processes. Any local authority not complying with the publications would have to justify why, and any specific local considerations that would vindicate any local variations. These documents are essential reading for any professional wishing to gain knowledge of the child protection processes according to the country in which they practise.

For ease of use, this book will refer to the simplified title that the publication for England and Wales is known by, which is *Working Together*. Any reference to *Working Together* will always be the publication mentioned in full above and should be assumed to also apply to the equivalent issue for Scotland, *Protecting Children*. Where the publications are different this will be made clear in the text. I would not wish Scottish colleagues to take offence; this is merely to avoid cumbersome usage for the reader.

This book begins by looking at the individual and social factors which influence how a mother relates to her unborn and newborn baby. It then focuses on the antenatal, intrapartum and postnatal care and support that midwives can give to families to maximize each woman's potential to mother her baby sensitively and with enjoyment. Some of the very early signs of an insecure attachment and bonding are explored. The ongoing chapters take the reader through the process and progress of the child protection procedures, moving from the initial referral stages and finishing with the legal system, including the courts. Case histories and how they were resolved are included throughout the chapters to illustrate the application of the theory in everyday practice, and should help with the understanding of the main text.

There may be terms used which are new to you and they may feel confusing; however, most of them will become easier to understand as you work your way through the chapters making sense of some of the complexities involved. By becoming familiar with the procedures you will become more confident when attending a child protection meeting, and your knowledge base will gradually be built up by dipping back into the book as an ongoing reference tool.

There can be no apology for reminding the reader that we are fortunate in our work as midwives; we are involved daily with families who are happy to welcome children into their lives, who bring up their children with success, mutual love and enjoyment. But let us not forget the task of those professionals who work with families at the thin end of the wedge – families that are less able, dysfunctional, chaotic or often hostile towards those who are doing their very best to perform a professional role in difficult circumstances.

Jenny Fraser
Norwich 2004

Acknowledgements

I am very grateful to many people for enabling the second edition of this book about child protection to be written, including Mary Seager, senior commissioning editor at Elsevier, who was aware of the need for an updated edition and gave constructive advice on the format. I am above all appreciative of Mary Nolan and her enthusiasm to become involved with the writing of this book. That enthusiasm passing on to me was the launch that I needed to get writing. I am very obliged to Mary for her valuable and worthwhile contribution in writing the first two chapters.

I am particularly indebted to three people for their wise advice and commitment to making sure that the information imparted is accurate and appropriate. The first is David Bloomfield, solicitor, who always makes the necessary time and space for me when it is needed; secondly, Tony McGhee, independent chair in Norwich, and finally Paul Howard, recently retired Police Inspector from the Norwich Family Protection Unit. Thanks must also go to Paul Howard for gallantly taking up the challenge of writing the Foreword for this book.

I need to acknowledge and give my thanks to Allan Fraser, who spent many hours of his well-earned retirement accessing information from the relevant people in his home town of Buckie in the north of Scotland, on my behalf. I also appreciate the hours he spent in the Elgin library, researching and acquiring first-hand knowledge of the Scottish system for my benefit and, ultimately, that of the readers.

The month in which I write these acknowledgements marks the publication of Lord Laming's enquiry into the death of Victoria Climbié. Lord Laming's report consists of a long list of recommendations to tighten up the child protection system. Lord Laming has proposed new national and local management structures regarding the protection of children. May the death of Victoria not be in vain – if child protection processes and procedures become more robust, with the ultimate aim of preventing untoward suffering for children in the future.

Finally, I would like to make reference to the daily pain and distress felt by Sean (not his real name), one of the case histories in Chapter 3, whose tragic experience gave me many sleepless nights. Within this scenario I want to acknowledge a policeman, Jim Blake, from the Family Protection Unit in Norwich, who painstakingly and doggedly built up the case against the perpetrator of Sean's suffering, culminating in a court appearance and a justifiable prison sentence for the culprit. May Sean spend some happy days free from fear in future, because of the actions taken by Jim. This is one child who has been protected by the child protection procedures and the world has become a safer place for him – there are many more children still out there in such need.

Jenny Fraser
Norwich 2004

Becoming a family: mothers, babies and fathers

This chapter looks at the principal factors which influence a mother's relationship with her newborn baby and her subsequent relationship with him as he grows up. It examines the concepts of bonding and attachment, and indicates what may happen if these processes are disturbed. Underpinning everything that is discussed is the recognition that:

- Each person (mother, baby, father) is unique
- Each couple is unique (mother/baby; father/baby; mother/father)
- Each family is unique.

Sophie is a thirty-four-year-old solicitor. She earns an excellent salary, drives a new car and holidays abroad. She has been married for 8 years to an overworked GP. Sophie is expecting her first baby, after several years of 'trying'. Her mother died 18 months ago and her father now lives abroad.

Janine is 17 years old. She works in a café at the large supermarket close to her flat. She has an on/off relationship with Jon who is not the father of her child. The father visits Janine occasionally and can be both verbally and physically aggressive. Janine knows that her own father is violent towards her mother. Her mother is highly protective towards Janine and very prepared to help with the baby.

EXPECTING A BABY AND PARENTS' EXPECTATIONS

Two women in very different circumstances. Both pregnant with their first baby. How easy will they find the transition to being a mother? You might identify certain 'risk' factors for both of them. Sophie and her partner have been DINKYS (dual-income-no-kids-yet) for a long time. She has a successful career that will have to be put on hold for a while. She has taken a long while to become pregnant so her pregnancy may be 'over-valued'. She appears to have little or no support from family members. Janine is young. Her relationship with her boyfriend is unsteady. Both she and her mother have suffered from domestic violence. You might consider that Sophie's financial and marital security will buffer her during the transition to motherhood, and that Janine's closeness to her own mother will help her, as women with high levels of social support appear to adapt to motherhood more easily (Younger, 1991; Grace, 1993).

Whatever their social and financial circumstances, both women are facing a 'major life crisis, a time of crucial psychological adjustment' (Percival & McCourt, 2000: 185). Advertising, sit coms, childcare manuals and parenting magazines which portray motherhood as 'ultimate fulfilment – exciting, pleasurable and rewarding, a positive experience' (Kent, 2000: 109) make it hard for women to have realistic expectations of what mothering will be like.

Of course, being a mother *is*, for the majority of women exciting, pleasurable and rewarding. Nonetheless, in the early weeks at least, it is also characterised by exhaustion. Exhaustion heightens the effect of physical complications following the birth, emotional upheaval and changes in relationships (Ruchala & Halstead, 1994). Sophie's and Janine's days may change from a daily round of work, household chores, eating and going out when they please to a timetable which is led by a person whose internal clock is not governed by adult routines.

Tulman et al. (1990) carried out an illuminating study of activities after childbirth. They asked women how quickly they achieved:

- their desired or required level of infant care responsibilities
- their usual level of household activities
- their usual levels of social and community activities
- their usual level of self-care activities.

At 6 weeks following the birth of their babies, fewer than 30% of the sample of 97 women had fully resumed their usual levels of either household, or social and community activities, and a quarter had still not got to grips with infant care activities. By 6 months, fewer than 20% had resumed the full range of their previous self-care activities. Yet in the UK, the 'maternal episode' is considered finished at 6 *weeks* postpartum. The woman has her postnatal check with her GP and provided that her uterus has fully involuted and her perineum has healed, she is discharged.

In medical terms (the terms usually applied) she has returned to her pre-pregnancy state. There is little leeway after this visit for women to be other than 'back to normal' in the view of health professionals, friends, employers or their own.

Many mothers and fathers living in twenty-first century Britain receive very little support as new parents. This is especially true of the majority ethnic group consisting of white Caucasians. The extended family is largely a thing of the past for this section of society. Grandparents and other relatives who are experienced parents no longer live close by to provide guidance and babysitting services, and to give the new parents practical and emotional assistance. Women from some ethnic groups still enjoy a traditional lying-in period to help them recover from the birth and give them time with their babies away from the demands of household tasks. However, many other women are expected to take up the reins of motherhood a few days after the birth, entertain guests come to admire the new baby, and then return to work at the end of a few months. It has been said that 'never before have mothers been asked to do so much for so many in return for so little!' (Sears, 1985).

Lack of support is compounded by women's heightened awareness of the importance of quality parenting, and fear of 'getting it wrong'. Anxieties about parenting start from the moment the baby is born. How quickly is it necessary to bond with the baby? If it isn't possible to hold the baby in the first hour of life, has opportunity of establishing a satisfactory relationship with him gone for ever? How often are those of us who work in maternity care bombarded with questions from anxious parents-to-be or new parents about what they can/cannot eat; whether the holes in the mattress should be at the top/bottom of the cot; how quickly their baby should be 'in a routine'? Every day there is a new scare in the papers about environmental dangers to pregnant women, or a new theory as to what causes cot death. Having a baby in the twenty-first century is certainly not a relaxed affair.

These are the pressures facing women whose domestic and social circumstances are reasonably good. For those living in poverty, eating a poor diet and experiencing substandard housing and basic facilities, the new pressures may weigh extra heavily on top of the old. Disadvantaged women may have reduced self-esteem and suffer from increased social isolation. These factors, in turn, are linked with habits such as smoking and alcohol abuse which further undermine health (Chadwick, 1994). When women are poorly nourished during pregnancy, their babies are predisposed to chronic illness in adulthood, such as hypertension, cardiovascular disease and diabetes (Martyn, 1994). People on below-average incomes are twice as likely to develop a mental illness as those on average and higher incomes. Although child abuse occurs in all strata of society, it is more likely to occur in families where there is no one earning a wage, and which are socially deprived. Two million children in Britain today live in workless households (www.poverty.org.uk).

Levels of domestic violence have reached epidemic proportions according to the Home Office (1999) which has published figures suggesting that one in four women will experience violence in their own homes at some point during their lives. The Home Affairs Select Committee of 1993 notes that domestic violence can take many forms, including physical assault, sexual abuse and rape, threats and intimidation, degradation, mental and verbal abuse, humiliation and systematic criticism and belittling. Women may be kept without money and in isolation. Victims of domestic violence are at risk of chronic physical and mental ill health, and of drug, alcohol and substance dependency. The children of women who are battered are also at risk of being abused, either by their mother's abuser or by their mother (Price & Baird, 2001). Domestic violence crosses the barriers of wealth and class. To understand its effects within the context of an affluent, middle class household, you might read Ruth Rendell's gripping novel *Harm Done* (2000):

And don't ask why she puts up with it, will you? Where can she go? Where can she take her children? She can't keep herself – at least, I suppose not – so who will keep her? And she doesn't tell people because, believe it or not, she's ashamed. *She's* ashamed. She dreads the neighbours knowing because *real* women, women who are beautiful enough and clever enough, and really good about the house, they don't get abused. (p. 313)

Domestic violence does not stop when women become pregnant. Evidence suggests that pregnancy often precipitates an escalation in violence, as the abuser seeks to impose control on a life which is currently beyond his reach. The 1994–1996 *Confidential Enquiry into Maternal Deaths* (DH, 1998) revealed that six women had been murdered by their partners. Pregnancy outcomes in situations of domestic violence are often poor, with women experiencing an increased rate of miscarriage and stillbirth and giving birth to babies who are very small for gestational age.

THROUGH LABOUR AND BIRTH TO PARENTING

A mother is in the making from the moment when a woman first realises she is pregnant, but labour and delivery are the principal components of her 'rite of passage', after which she is publicly recognised as a new mother. Penny Simkin's fascinating research (1992) shows how women in their sixties and seventies remember every detail of the days on which their children were born. There seems little doubt that women's feelings about themselves as women are significantly influenced by their experiences of giving birth:

Women strive to incorporate their labor and delivery experiences into their self-image as they form an identity as a mother. A woman's negative responses and dissatisfaction with the childbearing event may result in a lack of emotional health and negative perceptions of her newborn, thus impeding the development of maternal identity. (Fowles, 1998: 235)

The influence of labour and birth on the postnatal well-being of women and their attachment to their babies has been debated in the literature for many years. As early as 1980, Doering et al. (cited in Quine et al., 1993) alleged that the quality of a woman's childbirth experience was vital to her future relationship with her partner and her baby. In the 1980s, research explored whether there might be links between the use of obstetric technology and the subsequent emotional state of the mother. However, Ann Oakley concluded in 1990 that 'the findings of such studies are contradictory' (p. 45). Green et al.'s famous research, 'Great Expectations' (1988) argued that it was not what happened during birth, but women's feelings about what happened that counted, and that women's satisfaction with birth was related to how positively they described their babies. Importantly, Green found that this relationship was 'independent of both parity and class' (8: 20).

Midwives have sought to set up debriefing services for women following childbirth because they have recognised that women's feelings about themselves and their adjustment to motherhood are strongly influenced by the events of labour. What happens in the delivery room impacts on both the mother's physical and mental health. Kumar's analysis (1997) of 49 women's experiences of 'severe and extreme disorders of affection' found that difficulty in relating to the baby was significantly associated with 'recalled severe pain during labour and delivery' (p. 177). It is now generally accepted that post-traumatic stress disorder (PTSD) is not confined to people in war zones or those who have experienced major disasters such as the September 11th attack on the World Trade Center. PTSD is precipitated by any events which have involved excessive fear for life or bodily integrity, or for the life or well-being of a loved one, and may therefore be experienced by women following childbirth (Charles, 1997).

The medical model, which has defined women's experience of giving birth for the last 30 years, dangerously belittles the impact of what happens in labour on a woman's mental and emotional health. Obstetricians' agendas have focused on achieving a physically healthy mother and a physically healthy baby. For midwives, however, and for women and their families, this is only the tip of the iceberg. The events of labour and birth must be such that from the delivery room there emerges a mother whose self-esteem is high and who feels confident and competent to care for her baby; a birth companion – father, sister, grandmother or friend – who feels committed to the new family unit; and a baby who is allowed to manifest all the instinctive behaviour which promotes attachment between his mother and himself:

Disruption of maternal–infant interaction in the immediate postnatal period may set some women on the road to breastfeeding failure, and, possibly, alter their subsequent behaviour towards their children. (Enkin et al., 2000: 437)

Research (for example, Green et al., 1990; Fleissig, 1993; Stamp & Crowther, 1994) has repeatedly concluded that women's satisfaction with labour and birth is strongly related to their sense of being in control. Green et al. (1990) showed that the vast majority of women want to be in control of what doctors and midwives do to them during labour, and that what women want is relatively unaffected by education and parity (4: 5: 11). However, their study also revealed that women's expectations of whether they would be able to achieve what they wanted were strongly related to their educational and socio-economic status, with well-educated women expecting to have more control than their less privileged sisters.

The most vulnerable women, the women who have little or no power in their everyday lives, are those with the greatest need for control in childbirth. Women who have been the victims of sexual abuse may fear the process of giving birth as a re-enactment of past abuse. Parratt (1994) considers that while the need to trust carers, to have privacy and to feel secure are all important, the need for control predominates.

Women's self-esteem and self-confidence increase incrementally with their sense of being an equal partner with health-care professionals in decision-making. VandeVusse (1999) represents this correlation diagrammatically, as shown in Box 1.1.

Kirkham (1983) wryly questions whether putting women into the position of a passive patient and denying them information during labour is the best way of preparing them for the responsibilities and the day-to-day decision-making which constitute motherhood.

BONDING AND ATTACHMENT

The publication of *Birth and Bonding* by Klaus and Kennell in 1976 suggested that the early postpartum (days, even hours) was 'a "sensitive period" for the establishment of the "bond" between mother and child which, in turn, affected their long-term attachment and had extended consequences for their emotional well-being' (Crouch & Manderson, 1995: 837). Many changes in hospital practice were made as a result – mainly positive, but with some interesting limitations. Rooming-in gradually became the norm. The nurseries to which babies had been taken at night

---

BOX 1.1   Control of decisions (Based on VandeVusse (1999) Model of patterns of control and methods of decision-making related to emotions expressed in women's birth stories.)

JOINT: CAREGIVER AND WOMAN	WOMAN'S EXPRESSED EMOTIONS
Shared: through requests	confident, comfortable
Shared: through explanations	appreciative, honoured
Uncontested: through agreement	surprised, resigned
Contested: through adaptation	sad, angry, devalued
Contested: through refusal	unsettled, punished
UNILATERAL: CAREGIVER TO WOMAN	

so that their mothers could rest were closed, and women were encouraged to be far more actively involved in the care of their babies. Breastfeeding was promoted as the right way to feed a baby, although bottle feeding was just about OK. It was still not all right to take your baby into bed with you. In the delivery room, great emphasis was placed on the woman holding her baby as soon as he was born in the belief that there was a critical time for bonding. Since the 1970s, the findings of many studies have questioned the undue emphasis placed on the very early postnatal period and have concluded that:

Most mothers who are constrained from early contact with their babies, whether through illness, misguided hospital policies, or personal preference, are likely to overcome any effects of this separation in the longer term. (Enkin et al., 2000: 430)

Nonetheless, Enkin et al. (2000) conclude their summary of the immediate post-birth period by observing that practices which actively prevent the mother from getting to know her baby are certainly not permissible (p. 418). Simple common sense would suggest that the first meeting between mother and baby is likely to be highly significant. Kumar (1997) describes how most mothers feel a great surge of love for their new babies, but notes that between 15% and 30% 'experience transient delays in the onset of maternal affection' (p. 179). Women who have subsequently proved themselves to be loving and competent mothers have described a wide range of feelings when their babies were born. Some were so elated that they could not take their eyes off their babies, and others wanted only to sleep (Nolan, 1996: 189). Having a baby is like falling in love – some people are immediately attracted to each other, and others (perhaps the majority) find that love grows over a period of time. In the first days of life, a mother's feelings about her new baby wax and wane. She may doubt the wisdom of having had a baby. She may be fearful of her capacity to cope, and tearful when she contemplates the future. All of this, as any midwife knows, is perfectly normal. The common sense reality is that:

Frequently there is too much fatigue, discomfort and newness in the early days for love to flourish instantly. (Pears, 1993: 70)

The vast majority of mothers, however, will quickly manifest the typical behaviour of a woman who has bonded to her baby. She:

- devotes a great deal of time to her infant
- takes responsibility for his care and acts quickly in response to signals that he needs feeding or attention
- becomes rapidly confident in handling and soothing him
- enjoys being in close contact with him
- is patient with him.

The concept of attachment is derived from the work of John Bowlby (1971, 1975, 1981) which has been extremely significant for both health professionals and parents. Bowlby believed that babies and young children develop a kind of blueprint for the way that people relate to each other. This blueprint is based on the baby's experiences of being cared for by his mother. If the mother responds quickly and sensitively to his needs, the baby grows into a child who is trusting and affectionate. He sees himself as lovable, and is open to learning and life because he is confident that his basic needs will be met. If the mother ignores or misinterprets her baby's needs, the baby turns into a child who is frightened of being parted from her for fear that she may never return. He is mistrustful of other adults as well. He is either very demanding, or alternatively, withdrawn. Children with insecure attachment patterns are more at risk of being abused than their peers who are securely attached (Sydsjö et al., 2001). They appear to grow into adults who find it hard to form satisfying relationships with their own children.

Psychiatrists and psychologists think that attachment patterns are established by the time a child is 1 year old (Adams & Cotgrove, 1995). This is not to say that all is lost should the mother be 'unavailable' physically or mentally to her baby during that first year. Research has shown that babies can become attached to primary caregivers other than their mothers (Fonagy et al., 1994). Nonetheless, there are those who would argue that the loss of the relationship with the mother, even if *immediately* replaced by a relationship with a loving alternative carer, has an unavoidable adverse effect on the child (Verrier, 1996).

It might be thought that attachment is a two-way process – the baby attaches to the mother and the mother to the baby. Yet the evidence suggests that it is, in fact, the mother who plays the major role in the early development of attachment patterns. If the mother is depressed, suffering from drug addiction or oppressed by poverty and domestic violence, she may find it very hard to respond fully to her baby, and create the secure attachment that her baby needs (Sydsjö et al., 2001).

'DIFFICULT' BABIES AND GOOD MOTHERING

The pregnant parents' image of what their baby will be like is constructed on the basis of fantasy, ultrasound scans, media images, and comments made by relatives, friends and health professionals ('What a neat little bump!' 'This one's obviously a rugby player!'). Whatever the real baby looks like and however he behaves, he will undoubtedly be different from what the parents had imagined. There is also no doubt that some babies are more 'rewarding' than others. They are satisfyingly round and cuddly in appearance, and seem to be blessed from birth with cheerful personalities. Others are skinny, constantly demanding and to all intents and purposes, not at all pleased to have been born. Babies who feed five or six times a day, at fairly regular intervals and rarely at night, are termed 'good babies' (perhaps with the implication that their parents are 'good' parents?). Babies who want to suck at the breast or on the teat all the time and wake regularly during the night are termed 'difficult' or 'demanding' (with the implication that their parents have somehow got it wrong?). Mothers cannot be prevented from comparing their babies with those of other women, and guilt and confusion may set in if they feel that their baby's behaviour is a reflection on the quality of their mothering.

A 'difficult' baby certainly does not make the transition to parenthood any easier. However, there is no evidence that such babies fail to become securely attached if their mothers respond to their needs sensitively, or that they are the cause of postnatal depression. Difficult babies form normal attachments to their mothers provided that the mother is well supported during the time when the baby is particularly demanding. Mothers do not necessarily become depressed just because they have babies who cry a lot, although they may become very tired. The women who may find it difficult to respond appropriately to their crying babies and whose babies are therefore at risk of not becoming securely attached are those who have little support at home or in their wider social circle (Mills & Page, 2000). It is the woman's domestic and social circumstances, and her previous history of being parented, rather than her baby's temperament, that disable her mothering.

THE MOTHER'S EXPERIENCE OF BEING MOTHERED

No newborn baby is a blank script which parents can write on as they please, because genetics and the intra-uterine environment have been there before them. Equally, no new mother (or father) comes to parenting totally open-minded. The influences which make mothers mother in the way they do have been taking shape since they were themselves children. It would be wrong to say that there is no escape from either nature or nurture, but it would be wise to recognise the part they have played in moulding the clients whom we meet as prospective new parents. Most influential in the development of mothering skills is the woman's own experience of being mothered. Parenting style has been found to be a highly reliable indicator of children's well-being across a wide spectrum of environments, and whatever ethnic background the family belongs to (Darling & Steinberg, 1993). Women who have been 'undermothered', whose parents exhibited low responsiveness, were rejecting and/or neglectful are likely to have failed at school and to be unsuccessful in both the world of work and in relationships. Women who were physically or sexually abused as children are more likely to emotionally abuse their own children (Ney, 1988). Physical abuse and neglect, sexual abuse and psychological maltreatment may prove endemic in families, with health professionals and social workers witnessing a depressing recurrence of poor parenting from one generation to the next.

Nonetheless, it is important to recognise that people can be assisted to reflect on and learn the lessons of their past experiences. Parenting courses and family therapy depend on this premise. Grimshaw and McGuire's research (1998) shows how people can recognise and break the mould of parenting set in their own childhood. Following a parenting course, one father revealed that he had gained considerable insight:

I couldn't see anything else (any other way of fathering), because that was in my childhood, too . . . My father was violent towards us, as far as I can remember, and I feel that I was actually following a lot in his footsteps. (quoted in Nolan, 2002: 7)

In addition, important research rejects the theory that the early relationships are the only ones that count in the formation of parenting attitudes. Instead, a 'variety of vital relationships in the individual's life' seem to be influential 'in addition to the early care-giving relationship' (Mills & Page, 2000: 229). A relationship with a health professional may be significant in boosting a woman's self-esteem to the point where she is confident and competent to mother her own child.

PARENTING AND MENTAL ILLNESS

Women who are depressed after childbirth find it difficult to bond with their babies. The depressed mother is less likely to make body, eye or verbal contact with her baby than the mother who enjoys good mental health. She is less able to respond to the signals her baby sends out that he needs care and attention. She is less likely to be patient with her baby. These women are not poor mothers in the moral sense; they are poorly mothers.

People who are depressed have low levels of energy. The research of Tulman et al. (1990) informs us, not surprisingly, that women who have high levels of energy are able to resume their usual household chores, social life and self-care activities more quickly than those who have lower levels. Having no energy makes it harder to get out of the house to socialise with other women who have babies, and harder to maintain your own appearance and health upon which self-esteem is so dependent. People who are depressed withdraw into themselves – they struggle to meet their own daily needs, let alone those of others. The children of women who have suffered from or continue to suffer from postnatal depression display emotional and behavioural disturbances (Kumar, 1997).

It is difficult to predict which women will become depressed after childbirth, although it is known that women who were depressed during pregnancy are at high risk of postnatal mental ill health. It is commonly thought that the following factors predict depression:

- unwanted pregnancy
- significant health problems in pregnancy
- caesarean section
- general anaesthetic
- disappointment over gender of baby
- baby admitted to NICU
- problems with breastfeeding.

However, Kumar's research (1997) shows that this is not the case. Nor, according to Kumar, are women suffering from puerperal psychosis more likely than women suffering from non-psychotic illness to neglect or try to harm their babies. Women living in poverty and those struggling with drug addiction have a high risk of mental ill health and their children are at increased risk of turning into unhappy and disruptive youngsters. Boys seem to be more vulnerable to the effects of their mothers' mental illness than girls (Sydsjö et al., 2001).

FATHERS

Women without an extended family, and who lack support, are likely to depend very heavily on their partner. The popular press sometimes makes it hard for us to believe that the majority of fathers are still living in traditional family situations:

Four-fifths of dependent children still live in a family with two parents, and nine out of ten of those parents are married.
    More than eight in ten fathers still live with all their biological children, and more than seven in ten are doing so within their first family. (Family Policy Studies Centre, 2000)

This being so, there would seem to be a strong case for focusing more attention on fathers during pregnancy and the postnatal period and encouraging their support for new mothers. Research has shown that men still spend considerably less time with their babies and children than women, and that even when both partners are working full time, the mother continues to assume most of the responsibility for both the children's needs and household chores (Lamb, 1997). Yet men have stated that they want to be more involved in childcare.

    Health professionals and society at large may underestimate how little guidance there is available for new fathers.

Men are in a strangely ambiguous situation when it comes to impending fatherhood – expected to be more involved and caring but with little available to help them be so. (Jordan, 1990: 11)

    Fathers Direct, a new organisation concerned exclusively with the physical and mental well-being of fathers, finds that many men feel totally unprepared for parenthood. There is no specific role for fathers in our society to play during pregnancy, no set duties for them to fulfil. Men attending antenatal clinics with their partners may feel sidelined:

I was standing next to Karen, holding her hand. The midwife came along and said to her: 'Would you like to go along to the ultrasound department now. Tell your partner that he can go with you.' And this was while I was standing right next to her! (Alun: personal communication)

By contrast, in many traditional societies, men prepare for the birth of their child as wholeheartedly as their partners. Jacqueline Vincent Priya (1992) describes how fathers have to keep away from anything to do with death or dying as a means of protecting their baby against stillbirth. In Mexico, the father must not drink to excess, otherwise the baby may be weak, deformed or stillborn. In twenty-first century Western society, there still seems to be a tendency to expect men to provide the wages, pay the bills but otherwise, keep pretty much in the background. Yet men's involvement in childcare protects women against postnatal depression, enhances the relationship between the couple and leads to better parenting outcomes (Watson et al., 1995). Most men would like to be a central figure in their children's lives, but they may have few role models to guide them. Men may not have been fathered in the way that they would like to be fathers to their own children. In order to support their partners, men need support and preparation themselves. Where fathers are actively involved with their children, their children become more socially competent, are more successful at examinations at 16 and less likely to have a criminal record by the age of 21 (O'Sullivan: www.bbc.co.uk 7.11.01).

GRANDPARENTS

Women who do not have a partner or whose partner is abusive or unreliable are likely to turn to their families, especially their own mother, for emotional support, material assistance and help with the baby. After mothers and fathers themselves, the Family Policy Studies Centre (2000) notes that grandparents are the single most important source of pre-school childcare. Support from grandmothers may enhance the mother's educational and employment outcomes, but may have a more negative effect. Some research has shown that the babies of women with high levels of grandmother support form insecure attachments to their mothers, and the mothers themselves suffer from low self-esteem (Clement, 1998). Grandmothers may give advice which is destructive and belittling and find it difficult to get the balance right between supporting the mother and creating a non-helpful dependence in her which merely mimics the subservient position she may already endure in relation to her partner.

CONCLUSION

Whatever the circumstances of a mother or couple who have just become parents, however comfortably off they are, however well-educated, the transition to parenthood is never going to be an easy one. The gulf between expectations of what being a mum or dad will be like and the reality means that a considerable adjustment process is required after the birth of a baby. A mother's relationship with her baby will be influenced by many factors including her relationship with the baby's father, her socio-economic position, her educational background, her own experience of being parented, what happened during her labour and delivery, her mental health while she was pregnant and in the postnatal period and, above all, the degree to which she has the support either of her partner, or of significant others in her life who are able to encourage and praise her, and give her practical help with the multitude of tasks that need to be accomplished. Western society's expectations of when a woman should be 'back to normal' after giving birth are unreasonable, as are medical expectations which assume that the 6-weeks postnatal check marks the total restoration of the maternal body and mind to their pre-pregnancy state. In fact, for most women, it is months before they are able to give themselves and their social and working lives the degree of attention they had previously enjoyed.

The task of babyhood is to form a secure attachment with the mother or principal caregiver. This attachment would seem to depend far more on the mother's ability to understand and respond to her baby's cues than on the baby's temperament. Babies and mothers who are well attached to each other are far less likely than those who are insecurely attached to have traumatic relationships later on that involve abuse on the mother's part and disruptive behaviour on the child's.

The next chapter examines the vital part the midwife can play in promoting early attachment between mother and baby and in safeguarding the physical and mental health of the whole family.

ASK YOURSELF

1. Do you know where your local refuge for battered women is?
2. What aspects of care during labour are the most important for survivors of abuse?
3. Can you list four signs which indicate that a mother has bonded with her baby?
4. What factors may prevent a baby from attaching securely to its mother?
5. How do you attempt to incorporate significant members of the mother's family into her antenatal care?

REFERENCES

Adams L., Cotgrove A. (1995) Promoting secure attachment patterns in infancy and beyond. *Professional Care of Mother and Child*, 5(6):158–160.
Bowlby J. (1971) *Attachment and Loss. Volume 1: Attachment*. Harmondsworth: Penguin Books.
Bowlby J. (1975) *Attachment and Loss. Volume 2: Separation, Anxiety and Anger*. Harmondsworth: Penguin Books.
Bowlby J. (1981) *Attachment and Loss. Volume 3: Loss*. Harmondsworth: Penguin.
Chadwick J. (1994) Perinatal mortality and antenatal care. *Modern Midwife*, 4(9):18–20.
Charles C. (1997) When the dream goes wrong . . . post traumatic stress disorder. *Midwives*, 110(1317):250–252.
Clement S. (1998) *Psychological Perspectives on Pregnancy and Childbirth*. Edinburgh: Churchill Livingstone.
Crouch M., Manderson L. (1995) The social life of bonding theory. *Social Science and Medicine*, 41(6):837–844.
Darling N., Steinberg L. (1993) Parenting style as context: an integrative model. *Psychological Bulletin*, 113(3):487–496.
Department of Health (DH) (1998) *Why Mothers Die: Report on the Confidential Enquiries into Maternal Deaths in the UK 1994–1996*. London: HMSO.
Enkin M., Keirse M.J.N.C., Neilson J., Crowther C., Duley L., Hodnett E., Hofmeyr J. (2000) *A Guide to Effective Care in Pregnancy and Childbirth*. Oxford: Oxford University Press.
Family Policy Studies Centre (FPSC) (2000) *Family Change – Guide to the Issues – Family Briefing Paper 12*. London: FPSC.
Fleissig A. (1993) Are women given enough information by staff during labour and delivery? *Midwifery*, 9:7–25.
Fonagy P., Steele M., Higgit A. (1994) The theory and practice of resilience. *Journal of Child Psychology and Psychiatry*, 35:231–257.
Fowles E.R. (1998) Labor concerns of women two months after delivery. *Birth*, 25(4):235–240.
Grace J.T. (1993) Mothers' self-reports of parenthood across the first 6 months postpartum. *Research in Nursing and Health*, 16(6):431–439.
Green J.M., Coupland V.A., Kitzinger J.V. (1988) *Great Expectations: A Prospective Study of Women's Expectations and Experiences of Childbirth*, Volume 1. University of Cambridge: Child Care and Development Group.

Green J., Kitzinger J., Coupland V. (1990) Stereotypes of childbearing women: a look at some of the evidence. *Midwifery*, 6:125–132.

Grimshaw R., McGuire C. (1998) *Evaluating Parenting Programmes: A Study of Stakeholders' Views*. London: National Children's Enterprises Ltd.

Home Affairs Select Committee (1993) *Report on Domestic Violence*. London: Home Office.

Home Office (1999) *Domestic Violence: Break the Chains. Inter-departmental Guidance for Agencies Dealing with Domestic Violence*. London: Home Office.

Jordan P. (1990) Labouring for relevance: expectant and new fatherhood. *Nursing Research*, 39(1):11–16.

Kent J. (2000) *Social Perspectives on Pregnancy and Childbirth for Midwives, Nurses and the Caring Professions*. Buckingham: Open University Press.

Kirkham M.J. (1983) Labouring in the dark: limitations on the giving of information to enable patients to orientate themselves to likely events and timescale of labour. In: Wilson-Barnett J. (ed.) *Ten Studies in Patient Care*. London: John Wiley & Sons, 81–100.

Klaus M.H., Kennell J.H. (eds) (1976) *Maternal–Infant Bonding*. St Louis: C.V. Mosby.

Kumar C. (1997) "Anybody's child": severe disorders of mother-to-infant bonding. *British Journal of Psychiatry*, 171:175–181.

Lamb M. (ed.) (1997) *The Role of the Father in Child Development*. Chichester: Wiley.

Martyn C.N. (1994) Fetal and infant origins of cardiovascular disease. *Midwifery*, 10(2):61–66.

Mills B.C., Page L.A. (2000) The growth of human love and commitment. In: Page L.A. (ed.) *The New Midwifery*. Edinburgh: Churchill Livingstone, 223–244.

Ney B.G. (1988) Transgenerational abuse. *Child Psychiatry and Human Development*, 18(3):151–168.

Nolan M. (1996) *Being Pregnant, Giving Birth*. London: HMSO in collaboration with National Childbirth Trust Publishing Ltd.

Nolan M. (ed.) (2002) *Education and Support for Parenting*. Edinburgh: Baillière Tindall.

Oakley A., Rajan L. (1990) Obstetric technology and maternal wellbeing: a further research note. *Journal of Reproductive and Infant Psychology*, 8:45–55.

Parratt J. (1994) The experience of childbirth for the survivors of incest. *Midwifery*, 10:26–39.

Pears M. (1993) Love grows. *Midwives Journal*, 89(20):70.

Percival P., McCourt C. (2000) Becoming a parent. In: Page L.A. (ed.) *The New Midwifery*. Edinburgh: Churchill Livingstone, 185–221.

Price S., Baird K. (2001) Domestic violence in pregnancy. *The Practising Midwife*, 4(7):12–13.

Quine L., Rutter D.R., Gowen S. (1993) Women's satisfaction with the quality of the birth experience: a prospective study of social and psychological predictors. *Journal of Reproductive and Infant Psychology*, 11:107–113.

Rendell R. (2000) *Harm Done*. London: Arrow.

Ruchala P.L., Halstead L. (1994) The postpartum experience of low-risk women: a time of adjustment and change. *Maternal-Child Nursing Journal*, 22(3):83–89.

Sears W. (1985) *The Fussy Baby*. Franklin Park, IL: La Leche League International.

Simkin P. (1992) Just another day in a woman's life? Part II: Nature and consistency of women's long-term memories of their first birth experiences. *Birth*, 19(2):64–81.

Stamp G., Crowther C. (1994) Women's views of their postnatal care by midwives at an Adelaide Women's Hospital. *Midwifery*, 10:148–156.

Sydsjö G., Wadsby M., Göran Svedin C. (2001) Psychosocial risk factors: early mother–child interaction and behavioural disturbances in children at 8 years of age. *Journal of Reproductive and Infant Psychology*, 19(2):135–144.

Tulman L., Fawcett J., Groblewski L., Silverman L. (1990) Changes in functional status after childbirth. *Nursing Research*, 39(2):70–75.

VandeVusse L. (1999) Decision making in analyses of women's birth stories. *Birth*, 26(1):43–52.

Verrier N. (1996) *The Primal Wound – Understanding the Adopted Child*. Baltimore: Gateway Press.

Vincent Priya J. (1992) *Birth Tradition and Modern Pregnancy Care*. Element: Shaftesbury.

Watson W.J., Watson L., Wetzel W., Bader E., Talbot Y. (1995) Transition to parenthood: what about fathers? *Canadian Family Physician*, 41:807–812.

Younger J.B. (1991) A model of parenting stress. *Research in Nursing and Health*, 14(3):197–204.

2

Supporting parents and parenting

In order to nurture a child, a woman needs to feel valued and nurtured herself. She needs to have confidence in her own ability to think clearly and make good decisions for herself and her baby. The way parents are cared for during pregnancy and childbirth is crucial in laying down the foundations of confidence and self-esteem. (Schott, 1994: 3)

Midwives hold the potential to make a significant contribution to the health and happiness of mothers, babies and their families. (Page, 1995: 227)

Midwives' responsibility for preventing child abuse and family breakdown is fulfilled by helping every pregnant and new mother to bond with her baby as satisfactorily as possible. As well as monitoring the mother's physical welfare, there are a multitude of ways in which midwives can boost women's self-esteem and capacity to be 'available' to their babies. Parents with high self-esteem are able to rear children with high self-esteem. Dysfunctional families are those whose members have low expectations of themselves and others.

The previous chapter showed how the transition to parenthood has been viewed in the literature as a crisis. It is a crisis not just for the mother and father, but for the whole of society because the quality of parenting that our children experience determines the kind of citizens they will become. Percival and McCourt (2000) suggest that the new parenthood crisis is greater for women than for men. Midwives, who spend their time with pregnant women and new mothers, have the most wonderful opportunity to influence the transition to parenthood – for better or for worse. It is a heavy responsibility indeed.

Yet what women most want is not difficult to provide. They want to be treated kindly and with respect. They want their midwife to acknowledge just how enormous is the experience they are going through:

What is important is to give women the attention they deserve for the magnitude of the experience they are undergoing. (Peterson, 1993: 37)

This makes the issue of continuity of care a key one. In order to be able to understand how a woman is coping with the transition to motherhood, a midwife needs to get to know her, and her family, well. This does not mean that she necessarily has to be with the woman when she gives birth – although that would be ideal – but it does mean that she needs to be there for her in pregnancy and in the first weeks after her baby is born. Achieving as much continuity of *carer* (not just care) as possible from the antenatal to the postnatal period is one way of promoting the new mother's emotional as well as physical well-being.

Kindness is transmitted through verbal and non-verbal language. Women will interpret the midwife's body language to determine how focused she is on their needs and concerns (sitting down, leaning forward attentively or hovering in the doorway, ready to rush off to the next client? Touching her only for the purposes of the clinical examination, or putting an arm round her shoulders to nurture and encourage her?). Women listen to what their midwife is saying not only to gain information about their baby and their own state of health, but to gauge how well the midwife thinks they are carrying out the tasks of pregnancy and mothering. Comments on the size of the baby either in the woman's womb or in her arms will rarely be heard by the woman in the way the midwife intended! Being told that her baby is 'very big' or 'very small', or even simply 'big' or 'small' will keep a woman awake through the night. A comment that her baby 'is growing beautifully' and is 'just the right size' will have an effect on reducing her adrenaline levels out of all proportion to the remark itself.

IDENTIFYING WOMEN IN NEED: PROVIDING EXTRA SUPPORT

Listening visits

In the course of a relationship that spans the 9 months of pregnancy, a midwife will find out a great deal about which women on her caseload are going to find the transition to motherhood the most challenging. Antenatal clinics and home visits provide the midwife with a precious opportunity to identify mothers and families who may be at short- or long-term risk of social and emotional problems. In a more rational climate of care, these would be the women who receive more antenatal and postnatal visits, while women who are well supported would receive fewer. Ann Oakley's important research into providing social support in pregnancy for women from disadvantaged socio-economic groups clearly demonstrated that the effects of such support on the women, their children and their families are long-lasting:

Offering socially disadvantaged 'at risk' mothers additional support during pregnancy has a positive impact on measures of children's health status and family well-being 7 years later . . . perhaps most interesting of all is the fact that a number of conceptually different outcomes seem to be linked in the generally better outcomes of families offered pregnancy support. These include less maternal anxiety and fewer child accidents, better child development and sociability and increased male domestic participation. (Oakley et al., 1996: 20)

Oakley draws attention to the close relationship between physical health and social well-being, and argues that investing in extra support in pregnancy for selected women would result in cost-effective maternity services.

Clement's work (1995) has also focused on the importance of antenatal 'listening visits' to help women make a successful transition to motherhood. She feels that these visits must not stop at the end of pregnancy, but should extend into the postnatal period to 'ensure continuity of caregiver during the often critical period after birth when women may be feeling particularly vulnerable' (p. 77). Midwives' visits are often far more acceptable to vulnerable families than visits from a social worker whose care may be viewed as stigmatising. The midwife is seen primarily as providing health-related assistance, while the social worker's attention labels the family as 'at risk'.

Domestic violence

Midwives are perhaps more likely than any other group of professional workers to be able to find out if the woman is in an abusive relationship with her partner or with someone else in her family. Violence in the home is not restricted to families from poorer socio-economic groups, but affects all strata of society. A home in which women are abused is also likely to be a home where children are abused. Pregnancy is no guarantee of a woman's safety:

For some women, the pregnancy may act to trigger violence, for others it may result in an increase in existing patterns of abuse, possibly related to jealousy or anger towards the unborn child, or simply just 'business as usual'. (Price & Baird, 2001: 12)

The booking visit needs to include a carefully phrased question asking women whether there are ever occasions at home when they feel frightened or fear that they or their baby might be hurt. If women disclose that they are being abused, midwives need not feel that they have to take sole responsibility (Fraser, 2001), but it is important to be aware of the specialist professionals and voluntary organisations such as Women's Aid Outreach (see details at end of book) who can help.

Assessing parenting skills

It is very much easier to screen a pregnant woman for actual or potential physical problems that may affect the well-being of her baby, than it is to assess her parenting skills. Yet in terms of promoting the healthy functioning of families, helping a pregnant woman to understand her feelings about parenting and to assess her support networks is crucial. The previous chapter discussed how a woman's experience of being parented lays the foundations for her own style of parenting. Mills and Page (2000) describe a brief early pregnancy interview that the midwife can carry out to assess the woman's parenting history and her insight into its impact on her. They suggest questions such as:

- Could you tell me a little about your family when you were small?
- Which parent did you feel closest to and why?
- Could you describe how you were disciplined as a child?
- In what ways would you like to be like/not like your mother/father as you parent your child?
- Is there anything that you have learned from your experiences as a child? (p. 237)

It may be that questions such as these, asked by a sympathetic, known and trusted health-care professional will give a woman an opportunity to talk about her childhood that she has never had before. She may reveal a history of abuse with which she would like help so that she can address key issues about her own experience of being parented before she becomes a parent herself. Assessment of abusive families often reveals a multi-generational cycle of abuse. Abuse is thought to be twenty times more likely if one of the child's parents was abused as a child. Nevertheless, it is important to remember that more than a third of mothers who were abused either sexually, physically or emotionally as children are able to provide loving mothering for their own children (Meadow, 1997). The midwife can continue to explore parenting issues as the opportunities arise, or take advice on referring the woman for psychotherapy, counselling or mental health services. In her ongoing relationship with the woman, she can model nurturing behaviour by listening well, and providing support without criticising or giving advice. By doing this, she may be the first person who has ever made the woman feel good about herself.

MENTAL HEALTH IN PREGNANCY

Women of all ages and all cultures become depressed. Women with a history of depression are more likely to suffer from postnatal depression (Thorpe et al., 1992). Approximately two-thirds of women with postnatal depression were depressed antenatally. Only about 3% of women experience a first episode of depression following delivery (Glover, 2001). The signs of depression may be obvious – low mood, tearfulness, poor concentration, lack of energy, reduced or increased appetite, sleep problems and anxiety – but are often not so apparent because pregnancy can produce similar symptoms in women who are adjusting quite normally to their new situation. Depression may present not as emotional or psychological symptoms, but as physical complaints such as suffering from headaches, stomach problems or generalised aches and pains. Again, these kinds of problem are quite common in pregnancy and it can be hard to detect whether they are related to the woman's mental or physical health.

Difficult though it may be, checking the woman's mental health regularly during pregnancy by asking her whether she has any unusual feelings of not being able to cope, or of sadness or hopelessness, is worthwhile to detect those whose antenatal mood may persist into the postnatal period, and threaten their relationship with their new baby. Women noted as being depressed need extra monitoring and support after the birth to safeguard the functioning of the new family.

Good self-esteem is pivotal to mental health. The midwife can easily spot signs of low self-esteem. It is evident in the women who do not smile easily, who have a negative, hopeless view of themselves, their family and of society in general. They are unable to set themselves goals and prefer being alone to making the effort to meet other people. They avoid meeting you eye to eye, and have difficulty in trusting you. They fear adversity and do not want to take risks – life is already too risky. They may not tell the truth. They may demonstrate little compassion for others or remorse about actions they have taken which have hurt others.

Self-esteem results from a sense of mastery over life situations. Women from disadvantaged backgrounds may rarely experience such a sense of control. Their lives may be overtly or covertly controlled by others; they may be dependent on state benefits; they may feel out of control as a result of inadequate housing, difficulty in accessing services and the burden of debt. Feelings of incompetency at the threshold of motherhood place the woman at risk of depression. The midwife may not be able to change the woman's socio-economic circumstances, but she may be able to contribute to giving her some sense of mastery over becoming a parent. This can be assisted by inviting her to be an active participant in making decisions about her pregnancy and labour. She needs time to discuss her feelings about labour, and to have her hopes and fears validated as normal. She needs reassurance that there is no acceptable or non-acceptable way of behaving in labour and that she is entitled to cope with contractions in any way that she finds helpful. She needs to be informed that she has the right to ask for and expect respect, information and practical assistance from her caregivers in response to her physical and emotional needs during labour and after the baby is born. If the midwife is able to project a strong conviction that this woman can become a good mother, then she is promoting self-esteem and helping the woman to confront the challenges she faces. This does not mean expecting nothing of the woman – that is merely to express contempt for her abilities. Expecting her to be involved in thinking about her pregnancy and preparing for her baby helps build self-esteem and achievement. This is the kind of empowerment that a good set of antenatal classes would attempt to transmit, but women who are in the greatest need are rarely present at such classes.

Antenatal education currently reaches only a section of the childbearing population. Innovative ideas for reaching out to the people who currently do not attend classes are required. Women from disadvantaged backgrounds, who lack social support and have few skills for labour and parenting, are those who would especially benefit from classes. In working with women with little previous education either in a group situation or one-to-one, midwives have to devise opportunities for learning which take into account the following issues:

- There is no guarantee that clients have even elementary knowledge about their bodies.
- Clients may hold many beliefs about labour, babies and parenting based on incorrect or prejudiced information.
- Material must be presented in language that the clients can understand. (Many women, particularly working-class women, found the information given at classes difficult to remember and understand.) (Quine et al., 1993)

Pregnancy is a time when people are unusually open to looking at their lives and to making changes. It is regrettable that parent education is often given such a low profile in hospital and community services.

THE BEST LABOUR POSSIBLE

Recent research from Sweden (Persson & Dykes, 2002) showed how both women and men reacted negatively when the midwife presented herself as 'the expert' who dictates what is to happen and who does not expect to be challenged. When this attitude was replaced with one which acknowledged 'this is your birth, it is you who decide', both partners felt in control – with consequent positive effects on their emotional well-being.

Midwives play an important part in helping women embark on motherhood with enhanced confidence and self-esteem. They achieve this when they see women as capable of actively managing their birth experience, as opposed to patients whose reproductive system is unreliable, and requiring constant intervention (Moore & Hopper, 1995: 33). Page (1995) links the long-term future of the new family to the impact of care given during labour and birth:

The task of all professionals and particularly midwives is to give women and their families power around the births of their children. That personal power will help them in parenting over the many years that follow. (p. 231)

In order to cope with the stress and pain of labour, women need a range of personal and environmental resources which can be enhanced by the actions and responses of caregivers. Personal resources for coping are influenced by women's previous life experiences and especially their experiences of pain, and can be strengthened by empowering care from their midwives during pregnancy and labour. The environment where a woman gives birth sends out strong messages to her about whether it is she or others who are in control. The smells and sounds of the hospital, the delivery room where the bed holds centre-stage, the presence of monitoring and resuscitation equipment, all speak loudly to women that they are expected to assume a patient role. A hostile birthing environment can, however, be ameliorated by support. Bryanton et al. (1993) categorise support in labour under three headings:

- emotional
- tangible
- informational.

Emotional support involves reassurance and encouragement so that the woman gains a strong sense that there are people around her whom she can trust. Tangible support is holding, massaging and supporting the woman in the position of her choice, and providing physical comforts such as food, water, fresh clothes, ice-packs and warm compresses. Informational support means giving information freely, without its being requested, and making the woman feel that she is welcome to ask questions at any time, secure in the knowledge that she will receive full and honest answers. Even in emergency situations, Berg et al. (1996) found that:

Women wanted the staff to stop for just a second and communicate with them. Eye contact and explanation of the reason for interventions, followed by a moment of thinking, were desired in order to maintain the control and feel part of the birthing process. (p. 15)

Watson et al.'s recent research (1999) reports that, regardless of women's ethnic or cultural backgrounds, what they desire from, and appreciate in their caregivers during labour are clear explanations, the ability to listen and having their individual needs respected.

The absence of these attributes in a caregiver can make a relatively normal birth an unhappy experience or, conversely, a difficult birth may be perceived more positively if care has been sensitive and respectful. (p. 229)

Rowe-Murray and Fisher's study (2001) found that a low level of perceived support in labour and birth was significantly associated with greater mood disturbance in the early postpartum period. While women value encouragement and emotional and physical support during labour, it is known that professionals tend to spend very little time in providing this kind of care (McNiven et al., 1992).

Bick et al.'s overview (2002) of the field concludes that the presence of a loving support person in the delivery room is the best prophylactic against a woman's becoming postnatally depressed. This makes a strong argument for ensuring that whoever the woman chooses to have as her birth companion is an equal partner in intrapartum care. Not all birth companions will choose to adopt an active role in supporting the labouring woman, but many would like to help if shown what to do. Health-care providers can assist the woman's companions in identifying a role that is congruent with their personalities, their expectations and their relationship with the woman.

The midwife may not be able to remain with the woman throughout her labour; she can, however, assist the woman's chosen companion to provide active support in her absence. This, in turn, will promote the companion's self-esteem and enjoyment of the birth of the baby. Companions may be unsure about how to behave in the delivery room – eager for a role and yet terrified of doing something 'wrong'. The midwife can show them how to massage, breathe through contractions with the mother and help her into different positions. She can encourage them to offer comfort measures such as sips of water, bites to eat and warm compresses. Given a little guidance, the companion can be the midwife's strongest ally in enabling the woman to achieve a fulfilling birth.

Some women are especially needy in relation to labour and birth. About one in six is thought to suffer from an extreme fear of childbirth, called 'tokophobia'. This condition is not limited to particular age groups and crosses racial and cultural boundaries. Women report fear of pain, death and mental trauma, loss of control and lack of trust in the obstetric team. Sufferers describe their state of mind thus:

'I was convinced that I wouldn't survive the birth mentally, that I'd go mad with the pain.' (Jane: quoted in Hill, 2001)

'I had terrifying fantasies and images of childbirth.' (Laura: quoted in Hill, 2001)

There may be an increased risk of postnatal depression following the birth:

'I suffered postnatal depression and had real trouble bonding with my daughter . . . the whole experience was the most traumatic of my life.' (Laura, quoted in Hill, 2001)

These are women who may demand a caesarean section even when there is no obvious pathology in their pregnancies. They are likely to be well known to their midwives by the end and should ideally give birth in the care of a midwife known to them. Like all highly vulnerable women, they need constant reassurance during labour that they and their babies are fine, calm and detailed responses to their many queries, and support in confronting their fears. While it is easy to think that an epidural may be the answer to such women's difficulties, this is not necessarily the case as their mistrust of professionals and need to be in control may make the pain of normal birth more acceptable than agreeing to an intervention.

Pregnancy and labour are often major challenges for women who have been sexually abused during childhood. Although not often acknowledged in our society, sexuality, birthing and breast-feeding are all a part of women's psychosexual experience, and it is likely that 'childhood sexual abuse will negatively impact on birthing and breastfeeding, given its negative effects on sexuality' (Smith, 1993: 15). They find their bodies taken over by another person, and going through changes over which they have no control. A negative self-image may be made worse by the physical alterations of pregnancy. The experience of labour and birth, especially within a medicalised environment where multiple interventions are the norm, may reinforce active memories, or re-awaken dormant or suppressed memories of past abuse. Being on the receiving end of multiple intimate examinations in a brightly lit room filled with machines may intensify for the abused woman her previous experience of her body as an object 'manipulated' by others. Yet, she may be more at risk of interventions during her labour because the fear and tension caused by the situation increase the likelihood of dystocia. Survivors may use coping mechanisms to distance themselves from what is happening to them, which may also impede the course of their labours:

'I hadn't thought about the delivery in the sense of actually what was going to happen, but I had thought about my breathing . . . I think it was all up this part of me that I thought about. I didn't think about down there. Yes, that's where I concentrated – if I could keep that going on, then I'd be alright.' (quotation from Smith, 1993: 47)

This survivor endured a 56-hour labour by curling into a ball, obeying instructions from caregivers mechanically, and removing herself mentally from what was happening in her body and the delivery room. Little wonder that her labour lasted so long.

The midwife on delivery suite may or may not know that a particular woman has a history of abuse. The likelihood is that she will not. Indeed, the woman herself may not 'know' as she has repressed and 'forgotten' what happened to her as a child. Nonetheless, the midwife may pick up signs which could be indicative of previous trauma such as reluctance to be examined, abnormal levels of tension and distress, the woman trying to 'hide away' and protracted labour. Women appearing to be having such difficulties with labour need care which is sensitive to their exaggerated need for privacy, with careful attention given to the environment of birth, the language used to communicate with them and the number of carers whom they see.

BIRTH

The moment when a baby is born is the moment when the dynamics of nature (the baby's and mother's *instinctive* response to each other) and nurture (the mother's *conditioned* response to her baby) are at their most forceful. We rush in at our peril and are far better to adopt the part of the angels, fearing to intrude in this most critical period of the new family's life.

As the previous chapter has explained, there is no need for concern if the mother cannot spend the first minutes or even hours with her baby. However, if she can, so much the better. The surge of adrenaline which floods the mother's system in an unmedicated second stage prepares both her and the baby for the moment when they first meet. While caesarean section may unavoidably prevent early mother–infant interaction, in many cases it is hospital protocol and the rush to transfer the woman to the postnatal ward, rather than surgical delivery, which are the compromising factors. Research by Rowe-Murray and Fisher (2001) has shown that hospitals which adhere to the Baby

Friendly Initiative are more likely to encourage the mother to hold her baby as soon as possible after birth, than those which do not support the initiative. These researchers warn against making early mother–infant contact a 'psychosocial casualty of medically managed delivery' (p. 1073).

It may be that the woman who has just given birth is not going to keep her baby. Either the baby is going to be placed for adoption (although this is a decision that cannot be finalised for several months after the birth) or taken into care. In both these cases, it is still appropriate to encourage the mother to hold and interact with her baby. Whatever the mother's circumstances, whether the baby was wanted or not, the mother has been through the experience of pregnancy and birth, and giving up her baby will be a bereavement. Although a recent study (Hughes et al., 2002) has questioned accepted practice in the case of stillbirth of encouraging women to see and hold their babies, there remains a strong current of opinion that in order to facilitate grieving and subsequent mental health, the woman needs to know what she has lost and that this knowledge is best acquired through intimate contact with her child.

It may be tempting to avoid the woman who will not be leaving hospital with her baby because he is being taken into care. Doing so merely compounds her own opinion of herself that she is unfit to be a mother. Midwives need to be as available to her as to the other women on the postnatal ward whose circumstances are more 'ordinary'. It is important to allow the woman to express as much unhappiness as she is feeling and is willing to share. Carers may feel a deep sense of helplessness, but this should not prevent them from reaching out. Making comments about how the woman should or should not be feeling, changing the subject when she mentions her loss, pointing out that there are certain things she should be grateful for, will only serve to compound the feelings of self-doubt and guilt with which she will doubtless be struggling.

IDENTIFYING AND SUPPORTING VULNERABLE MOTHERS IN THE POSTNATAL PERIOD

While there are various tools which can be used to assess the quality of a mother's interactions with her baby in the early days of life, it is unreasonable to expect busy midwives working on understaffed postnatal wards to administer such tools to every woman who stays for just 2 days. Nevertheless, by carefully

observing the women in their care, ho.
of unease between mother and baby and
tion on to community midwives. Postnat
increased or their focus changed so as to pre
and support to help the mother who is finding .
act with her baby.

Midwives can assess the mother/baby relations. ....rv-
ing the extent to which the mother engages in t. ...owing
behaviours:

Close contact: holding the infant in close contact with her body,
clothed or unclothed, and encircling him with an arm as much
as possible.

Eye contact: attempting to make eye contact with her baby, even
if unsuccessful; placing him face to face.

Loving touch: touching the infant lovingly – gently stroking, kiss-
ing, patting and caressing him.

Examining the infant: lifting the blanket to look at the infant,
opening his hands to inspect the fingers, examining the feet,
etc.

Loving talk: talking lovingly to the baby, where 'lovingly' refers
to both affectionate tone and content.

Positive comments: making positive comments about the infant,
either descriptive (using, for example, adjectives such as *pretty*,
good, *beautiful*, etc.) or projective about the future ('You're going
to be such a pretty girl when you grow up').

Happiness: smiling and/or appearing happy >75% of the time.
(Based on Britton et al., 2001: 909.)

While such signs may not always be reliable in predicting the
future quality of the mother's relationship with her child, common sense would indicate that women who take active pleasure
in their new babies are off to a good start in their mothering.

TARGETING VULNERABLE FAMILIES

Providing extra support to vulnerable families in the early weeks
and months of parenting appears to have a favourable effect on
the quality of maternal–infant attachment. Bornstein (1995) con-
tends that mothers require supportive relationships with 'secondary parents' in order to sustain the emotional demands of
parenting. Health professionals who see the mother regularly,

who encourage, reassure her, and build her self-esteem, can act as the 'secondary parent' that she needs. Armstrong et al. (2000) compared 80 families who were randomly assigned to receive a series of weekly and then fortnightly visits from a child health nurse until the baby was 3 months old, with 80 who were invited to attend the child health clinic but did not receive special visits. At 4 months, the intervention families demonstrated enhanced maternal–infant attachment. The babies sustained fewer injuries and bruising and their mothers felt more competent and fulfilled as parents. The authors note that for many participants in this study, being a successful parent was seen as the first major positive achievement in their lives.

While all women need and deserve support in the postnatal period, it would seem a rational deployment of limited resources to concentrate on those families with known risk factors or where the early interactions between mother and baby in the delivery room and on the postnatal ward have given cause for concern. There are various ways in which the midwife can help maximise the mental health and functioning of the new family. The first of these, the most obvious and perhaps the most overlooked, is simply to listen to the mother. Mauthner (1997) notes that women want the opportunity to talk through their feelings about motherhood, both positive and negative, with someone prepared to listen to them non-judgementally. They want reassurance that their feelings are the same as those of other women. Clement (1995) suggests that were midwives to provide 'listening visits' for women until the end of the first postnatal month, they would be better able to detect the early signs of depression and make the appropriate referrals. While the Edinburgh Postnatal Depression Scale is a useful tool for detecting women at risk of or experiencing postnatal depression, Clement emphasises that it is not intended to replace or displace personal contact with the mother.

Fathers

If women have a steady partner or husband, it is vital to include them in the care of the new family, helping them to acquire practical babycare skills, and responding empathically to their uncertainties as they make the transition to fatherhood. This applies even and especially to fathers who, in the midwife's opinion, may not seem very promising as supporters of either their partner or their child. A study carried out at Newcastle University (Speak et al., 1997) interviewed single, non-resident, non-custodial fathers aged between 16 and 24. These young men did want to be involved with their children, many expressing the desire to be a different kind of father from their own fathers who had exhibited bad or abusive behaviour towards their offspring. The study found that disadvantaged young men were made to feel unimportant both before and after the birth and no encouragement was given to them to be involved with their baby, despite their keenness to 'be there'. The young mothers did not recognise the importance of fathers being involved with their children and sometimes rejected help from them when it was offered. Yet the young men did not feel it was beneath their manhood to change nappies, feed and bathe babies, and were occasionally willing to babysit so that the mother could have a little time to herself. While most of the young men were not contributing financially towards their child's maintenance, they did offer gifts, clothing, treats and practical childcare when cash was limited.

The researchers concluded that all those involved in the care of young families need to understand the role that fathers can play, and the factors that help or hinder their positive involvement with their children. If fathers are willing to be supportive, they should be shown how to help, encouraged and praised as in the case of any other father who might appear to be more promising material in terms of providing support for mother and baby.

Grandparents

Women who cannot call upon a partner for practical and emotional assistance in the early weeks of their babies' lives will naturally turn to their own mothers to fill the gap. By supporting grandmothers to support mothers, midwives can have a twofold effect – boosting the grandmother's self-esteem and protecting the mother's mental health.

The support that is provided in the early weeks of parenting is vital to the future well-being of the woman and her baby and family. It is no longer considered that the only relevant relationship in which the baby is engaged at this time is with his mother. The baby is affected by and affects a network of relationships extending beyond his mother (Adams & Cotgrove, 1995). Postnatal visits are an opportunity to nurture the family, however that is constituted, listening to the concerns of each member, and ensuring that each is aware of how to make the home environment a place where the baby can achieve optimum physical and mental development.

Where a mother has no one to support her, she may like assistance from one of the voluntary organisations concerned with families. Organisations such as *Homestart*, *Gingerbread* and the *National Childbirth Trust* can provide postnatal support on a one-to-one basis and the opportunity to meet other mums beyond the time when the midwife's contact with the mother ceases.

CONCLUSION

Every encounter between the mother and the midwife from the start of pregnancy until the end of their relationship between the 10th and 28th day following the birth of the baby, is an opportunity for the midwife to support the woman through the transition to parenting, and to safeguard the healthy functioning of the new family. To be able to provide effective emotional and psychological support, women need to see the same midwife or a small group of midwives throughout the maternity episode. The midwife who knows her clients well can identify women at risk of not bonding with their babies and the babies in turn forming insecure attachments to their mothers. She is the professional most likely to spot the pregnant woman who has mental health problems, the person in whom the abused or frightened woman may confide. She can develop a relationship in which it is possible for the disadvantaged mother to explore the influences that will affect her ability to nurture her new baby, and understand new ways of being a mother so as to break the cycle of inadequate parenting of which she may be a victim. By going beyond the clinical examination to *being with* women through the crisis of new motherhood, the midwife may be able to prevent later family dysfunction. Even one child saved from abuse is an achievement worthy of a lifetime in the profession.

ASK YOURSELF

1. Does the antenatal care you provide include an opportunity for the woman to talk about her experiences of being mothered?
2. Can you list six signs of depression?
3. To what extent does the care you provide during labour encompass emotional and physical support for the woman?
4. On your postnatal ward, does the woman who is not going to keep her baby receive the same level of recognition that she is a mother as other women?
5. Does the postnatal care you provide include significant members of the woman's family or support network?

REFERENCES

Adams L., Cotgrove A. (1995) Promoting secure attachment patterns in infancy and beyond. *Professional Care of Mother and Child*, 5(6):158–160.

Armstrong K.L., Fraser J.A., Dadds M.R., Morris J. (2000) Promoting secure attachment, maternal mood and child health in a vulnerable population: a randomized controlled trial. *Journal of Paediatrics and Child Health*, 36(6):555–562.

Berg M., Lundgren I., Hermansson E., Wahlberg V. (1996) Women's experience of the encounter with the midwife during childbirth. *Midwifery*, 12:11–15.

Bick D., MacArthur C., Knowles H., Winter H. (2002) *Postnatal Care: Evidence and Guidelines for Management*. Edinburgh: Churchill Livingstone.

Bornstein M.H. (1995) Parenting infants. In: Bornstein M.H. (ed.) *Handbook of Parenting. Volume 1: Children and Parenting*. New Jersey: Lawrence Erlbaum Associates, 3–39.

Britton H.L., Gronwaldt V., Britton J.R. (2001) Maternal postpartum behaviors and mother–infant relationship during the first year of life. *Journal of Pediatrics*, 138(6):905–909.

Bryanton J., Fraser-Davey H., Sullivan P. (1993) Women's perceptions of nursing support during labor. *Journal of Obstetric, Gynaecological and Neonatal Nursing*, 23(8):638–643.

Clement S. (1995) 'Listening visits' in pregnancy: a strategy for preventing postnatal depression? *Midwifery*, II(2):75–80.

Fraser J. (2001) Carly is sixteen. *The Practising Midwife*, 4(7):20–21.

Glover G. (2001) *Antenatal and Postnatal Mood: The Effects on the Fetus and the Child*. Proceedings of the First Conference of the Community Practitioners and Health Visitors Association (CPHVA) Postnatal Depression and Maternal Mental Health Network, 22 June. London: CPHVA, 13–15.

Hill A. (2001) Extreme fear of birth pain forces women to miscarry. *The Observer*, 16 December.

Hughes P., Turton P., Hopper E., Evans C.D.H. (2002) Assessment of guidelines for good practice in psychosocial care after stillbirth: a cohort study. *The Lancet*, 360:114–118.

McNiven P., Hodnett E., O'Brien-Pallas L. (1992) Supporting women in labor: a work sampling study of the activities of labor and delivery nurses. *Birth*, 19(1):3–8.

Mauthner N.S. (1997) Postnatal depression: how can midwives help? *Midwifery*, 13:163–171.

Meadow R. (1997) *ABC of Child Abuse*, 3rd edn. London: BMJ Publishing Group.

Mills B.C., Page L.A. (2000) The growth of human love and commitment. In: Page L.A. (ed.) *The New Midwifery: Science and Sensitivity in Practice*. Edinburgh: Churchill Livingstone, 223–244.

Moore M., Hopper U. (1995) Do birth plans empower women? Evaluation of a hospital birth plan. *Birth*, 22(1):29–36.

Oakley A., Hickey D., Rajan L., Rigby A. (1996) Social support in pregnancy: does it have long-term effects? *Journal of Reproductive and Infant Psychology*, 14:7–22.

Page L. (1995) Change and power in midwifery. *Birth*, 2(4):227–231.

Percival P., McCourt C. (2000) Becoming a parent. In: Page L. (ed.) *The New Midwifery: Science and Sensitivity in Practice*. Edinburgh: Churchill Livingstone, 185–221.

Persson E.K., Dykes A.K. (2002) Parents' experiences of early discharge from hospital after birth in Sweden. *Midwifery*, 18:53–60.

Peterson G. (1993) An easier childbirth. *International Journal of Childbirth Education*, 12(1):36–37.

Price S., Baird K. (2001) Domestic violence in pregnancy. *The Practising Midwife*, 4(7):12–13.

Quine L., Rutter D.R., Gowen S. (1993) Women's satisfaction with the quality of the birth experience: a prospective study of social and psychological predictors. *Journal of Reproductive and Infant Psychology*, 11:107–113.

Rowe-Murray H.J., Fisher J.R.W. (2001) Operative intervention in delivery is associated with compromised early mother–infant interaction. *British Journal of Obstetrics and Gynaecology*, 108:1068–1075.

Schott J. (1994) The importance of encouraging women to think for themselves. *British Journal of Midwifery*, 2(1):3–4.

Smith P. (1993) *Childhood Sexual Abuse, Sexuality, Pregnancy and Birthing: A Life History Study*. Manchester: PCCS Books.

Speak S., Cameron S., Gilroy R. (1997) *Young Single Fathers: Participation in Fatherhood – Bridges and Barriers*. London: Family Policy Studies Centre.

Thorpe K.J., Dragonas T., Golding J. (1992) The effects of psychosocial factors on the mother's emotional well-being during early parenthood: a cross-cultural study of Britain and Greece. *Journal of Reproductive and Infant Psychology*, 10:205–217.

Watson L., Potter A., Donohue L. (1999) Midwives in Victoria, Australia: a survey of current issues and job satisfaction. *Midwifery*, 15(4):216–131.

3

When to trigger child protection procedures and what happens following a referral

The previous two chapters have focused on the transition to parenting, and ways in which midwives can support women and their families as they face new challenges in their lives. The subsequent chapters will focus on families at the thin end of the wedge; those families who find that their capacity to parent, for many different reasons, is severely limited – resulting in children becoming compromised. Families without the capacity to care for their children adequately, or safely, may find that they become caught up in child protection procedures. Midwives have a crucial part to play in protecting children and a midwife needs to know what is involved within the child protection process, and how her role sits within it. In these circumstances it is vital that the midwife becomes familiar with the statutory framework that protects children.

The midwife must therefore have knowledge of the current legislation regarding the protection of children and her responsibilities towards a child in need of protecting. The minimum knowledge necessary must be:

• Know where your local area child protection committee (ACPC) manual is held for midwives working in England and Wales and where your local child protection committee (CPC) manual is held if you are a midwife working in Scotland.

• Have a working knowledge of what is contained within these manuals.

• Know whether you can access child protection policies and procedures on your intranet.

• Know your local policy for triggering child protection procedures.

• Have information about 'Working Together' if a midwife in England or Wales or 'Protecting Children' if a midwife working in Scotland, and the expectation of sharing responsibility regarding the protection of children by working with other agencies.

• Know who the named professionals for child protection are within your acute trust or primary care trust (PCT) if working in the community.
• Know who the designated nurse and doctor for child protection are within your health authority.
• The ability to recognise the signs and symptoms of child abuse.

The very nature of a midwife's work places her in a position whereby a close view of the family is seen. The midwife therefore is uniquely placed to identify risk factors to the child during pregnancy, birth and the child's early care (DH, 1997).

WHY YOU SHOULD KNOW ABOUT CHILD PROTECTION

It is vital that midwives recognise families in crisis and children in need, as the long-term effects of abuse on children can have untoward ramifications, which can last all their lives. These children in turn find it difficult to parent their own offspring and a vicious circle of inadequate parenting and subsequent further damaged children is maintained, which can affect the very fabric of our society. In addition, all children have the right to a safe and happy childhood.

Child protection procedures are lengthy, complex and expensive – both in monetary terms and human cost, upsetting and unsettling for the families and often the professionals involved. However, child protection measures are an absolute necessity if a child is deemed to be in danger. Midwives, of course, work with particularly vulnerable children, as babies are completely dependent on their carers for all their needs and cannot survive without those needs being met. The previous chapter described some of the ways in which midwives can support women and their families to be good enough parents, and some of the individual and social challenges that might make it difficult for mothers to respond appropriately to their babies' needs.

Midwives can miss child protection concerns within families, as this aspect does not form the usual bulk of midwifery work. It is different if the problem has already been highlighted, but recognising problems not already indicated might make you doubtful about what you are seeing. It is important to keep your eyes and ears open and to always seek advice and help from the relevant professionals, if you are concerned. This can help you to process your thoughts, enabling you to think more clearly and objectively.

Early detection of families at risk, from whatever source, and the subsequent instigation of timely support and care, may be enough to offset the need to activate child protection procedures. All families find themselves in difficult circumstances at some point in their lives, but some families have the capacity to cope with added burdens better than others. Having a baby in itself is a major life event and becoming a parent is probably the most demanding job ever undertaken in a lifetime. The way a mother adjusts to this new status is influenced by several factors: the quality of her own experience of being mothered, her personality, her experience of childbirth dovetailed with her conjecture of childbirth and her expectations of her baby and of being a mother. In addition to having a baby, if a mother has an extra burden such as poverty, domestic violence/abuse, homelessness or some other major difficulty, then she is highly likely to need some enhanced support in order to be able to care for her baby adequately. Babies need to have at least one parent or carer with adequate parenting capacity in order for them to thrive, thus enabling them to grow up feeling confident and happy in the world.

If a family in your area is very burdened, then taking some of the pressure off may help, until the family find themselves on an even keel again, thereby restricting the spilling over of emotions onto their children.

With some exceptions midwives are welcomed into families and so they can absorb a unique view of the family dynamics. Families do not generally see midwives as a threat, they talk to us, tell us their innermost fears, anxieties and worries. If you notice a family that is struggling, either emotionally or practically, your local knowledge of support groups or help available may improve the situation. The family may live in a Sure Start area, which would be an ideal early contact.

RECOGNISING CHILD ABUSE

This list is for general guidance only and is not meant to be exhaustive. The midwife should be alerted to possible potential problems in any of the following circumstances:

- Bruising or other injuries with no adequate explanation.
- A torn frenulum without an adequate explanation. In accidental circumstances the parents would seek immediate medical care.
- Grasp marks or fingertip bruising.
- Unexplained fractures.
- Scalds.
- Burns, particularly cigarette burns in unusual areas, such as the sole of the feet in a non-mobile child.
- Any delay in seeking medical advice.
- Vague history that lacks detail and is inconsistent when repeated.
- History of shaking.
- Parents' inappropriate reaction to the injury, i.e. not appearing particularly concerned.
- Bites, either human or animal.
- Neglect of basic physical needs, such as hygiene or feeding.
- Where the parents are fabricating an illness in their baby or child, causing medical tests to be carried out on the child, that are not necessary.
- Unrealistic expectations of the baby or child.
- Blaming a baby for apparent untoward behaviour; for example, blaming the baby for the pain felt during the birth or claiming that the baby has soiled its nappy on purpose in order to irritate its parent.
- Making undermining comments to a baby even though the baby cannot verbally understand, such as, suggesting the baby is ugly or has a bad temper. Such comments will invariably continue as the baby grows older, unless successfully contested with adequate explanations that are understood and acted upon by the parents.

WHEN AND HOW TO TRIGGER CHILD PROTECTION CONCERNS

Your starting point would be that in the course of your work you suspect that a child is suffering from or likely to suffer significant harm. Dimond (2002) says that to make a diagnosis of child abuse is a weighty matter. This is indeed true and the ramifications of disclosure of such suspicions can be enormous. 'Working Together' says: 'the difficulties of assessing the risk of harm should not be underestimated. It is imperative that everyone who deals with allegations and suspicions of abuse maintains an open and inquiring mind'.

It is important to take note that the above paragraph does not preclude you taking action about any child within the family, and does not limit your powers of observation to the baby, whether born or unborn. An example of this is illustrated in Case history 3.1. In this scenario the midwife realised that she was, in all probability, seeing a child that was a victim of a physical assault. It would not be in the public interest, and certainly not in the child's best interests to take no action.

Case history 3.1

Sonia's community midwife visited her two days postnatally at home. Sonia had given birth to her third child normally, in hospital, in the early hours of the previous day. She arrived home the previous evening at approximately 20.00 hours, about 16 hours after the birth. The midwife had a student midwife with her for this visit and on arrival Sonia was seated on the sofa holding her baby. Chris, her partner, was in the kitchen giving Sonia's two boys, both from different previous relationships, some breakfast. The midwife had never met Chris before as Sonia had always attended antenatal appointments alone. The eldest boy, Sean, was 6 years old and the younger boy David was 4 years old.

Sean finished his breakfast and came through into the lounge where his mum and the midwife and student were sitting. It was immediately obvious to the midwife that Sean had extensive trauma to his face. He had a new black eye, evidence of old bruising on his face and a massive large bump on his forehead. The midwife asked Sean how he had hurt himself and he replied that Chris had hit him and thrown him against the windowsill. While Sean was relating his story Sonia tried to speak over him to try and drown out the information that Sean was giving. Meanwhile Chris darted into the lounge shouting loudly at Sean and demanded that he went to his room. He stood menacingly over Sean until he eventually did as he was told. David was noted to be cowering quietly in the kitchen.

On leaving the house the midwife said to both Sonia and Chris that she would have no alternative but to inform her manager and social services about what she had seen and heard.

The midwife and student left the house and parked the car nearby in order to verify what they had heard. They wrote the conversation down should the information be needed at a later stage. Social services were duly informed and they reacted immediately by visiting the house and taking Sean to a paediatrician for an examination. The paediatrician felt fairly certain that he was seeing a child with a non-accidental injury.

Continued

Case history 3.1—cont'd

Background enquiries revealed a child that was subject to many concerns. A strategy discussion took place without delay the same day, over the telephone, and a child protection conference was swiftly convened the following day. During the child protection conference Sean's teacher described how Sean regularly had bruises or burn marks on a daily basis and that she had profound concerns about Sean's safety. This teacher was also concerned that Sean would often not be at school and when questioned Sean would say that he was ill; however, these episodes coincided with obvious physical trauma that had taken place. It seemed apparent that if Sean were particularly bruised, or had other significant marks, then he would be kept away from school until these were resolving. The conference decided that Sean's name should be entered onto the child protection register under the category of physical abuse.

Chris was taken to a police station for questioning about the injuries received by Sean. Sean though remained living at home with his mum and Chris with support from social services.

It was several months later that Sean was eventually removed from home into foster care, as despite the support into the home environment the abuse continued unabated. Sean missed his mother in foster care but despite this he flourished and started to have some of his daily fears of physical abuse removed. Sean was well supported at school and had a teacher that he particularly liked and little by little began to improve educationally.

A criminal conviction was pursued on Chris and ultimately he was summonsed to appear in court. The police had taken statements from the midwife and student and the original piece of paper used to write details of the original conversation down was used in evidence. The midwives were asked to attend court as witnesses, but Chris decided to plead guilty and therefore the midwives' oral evidence was not needed. While the police were pursuing this criminal conviction, the allocated police officer from the specialist unit which deals with child protection made regular visits to Sean to ascertain his views about his future. In time, Chris was convicted of cruelty and received an 18-month custodial sentence for the crime.

The midwife within this situation followed her local guidelines for the correct referral route. She took advice initially from her line manager who suggested that she contact the named midwife for child protection, and this she did. Within the health services there are individuals who have particular child protection responsibilities. These individuals are named child protection professionals. It is important that you are aware of the named individuals within your trust. The grave circumstances within this scenario warranted an immediate referral to social services and the named midwife supported the midwife through this action.

Any communication you have between yourself and your line manager or named midwife/nurse for child protection is a legitimate interchange between professionals and such help should always be accessed.

You must always remember that you have a duty to express your concerns to the appropriate people if you have concerns about an unborn baby or child that you have contact with. You have a clear responsibility to protect a child from harm. You are professionally accountable and responsible for your practice and actions or inactions.

At some point, if the concerns are severe enough, a referral will be made to a statutory agency, which is normally social services. This may be made by telephone or, if not immediately urgent, a written application. It is usual that specified referral forms for such circumstances are used for a written referral, and these need to be available to you. You will need to know where these can be accessed and you will possibly need some guidance when completing the form, before sending it. It is sensible to use colleagues who have specialist knowledge in child protection procedures to guide you; it can save a lot of time in the long run if the written referral is filled in correctly at the beginning.

Except in exceptional circumstances a referral should not be made to a statutory agency without the parents' knowledge, or before they have had the opportunity to listen, digest and discuss the concerns. This is good practice that will hopefully mean that the family is more likely to co-operate with the procedures, and lessens the chance of the family becoming hostile towards the process and the workers involved.

'Working Together' says: 'Parents' permission should be sought before discussing a referral about them with other agencies unless permission seeking may itself place a child at risk of significant harm'. In other words while it is good practice to inform parents, parental permission is not obligatory where it is felt that a child has suffered or is likely to suffer significant harm. Apart from these situations, in most circumstances, parents would be informed in advance of a referral being made. Any written referral should make it clear whether or not the parents have been informed.

As previously mentioned the most common route for a referral initiated by the midwifery services would be to a duty social worker employed by the local authority; however, a referral can also be made to the NSPCC or the police, according to the circumstances. A professional or a member of the public can make a referral. Your referral can be urgent where the child is in immediate danger, or less immediate when instant 'on the spot' decisions do not have to be made and a more thorough investigation of the issues can be commenced.

The police have immediate powers, which are discussed in Chapter 7, and their help may be needed in an acutely dangerous situation. The statutory powers of the NSPCC are also discussed in Chapter 7. The child protection process follows the same route, whichever agency is the first point of contact. All the agencies are expected to co-operate together and to communicate effectively, so that all the differing roles and responsibilities fall into place to safeguard the child.

WHAT HAPPENS FOLLOWING A REFERRAL?

There is an expectation that any referral from a professional to the agency with statutory powers will have carefully considered the information and gathered some background information before making the referral. This would be the same whether the baby was unborn or born. There are certain processes that should be undertaken in either scenario. They are:

- If working in the community this could involve speaking to the family's health visitor and GP.
- If working in hospital it is worthwhile communicating with the community midwife who in turn will access information as above.
- Discuss who will speak to the appropriate senior staff with specialist child protection experience, be this your manager or the named midwife or nurse. This background information will give her a fuller picture and she will then be in a better position to advise you.
- If you have any doubts as to whether this is a case of child protection or not then speak to the appropriate individuals anyway. Do not keep quiet about any concerns, no matter how seemingly trivial to you, if there is any chance that this could be a need for a child to be protected.
- Decide, with the appropriate support, by whom and how this information will be relayed to the family in question. Do not be

tempted to jump in and talk about a referral to social services with the family, unless obvious immediate protection is necessary, until you have fully discussed the situation with the appropriate people. Under no circumstances should you place yourself in any danger from a family; get suitable advice. In exceptional circumstances where a child could be put at further risk following disclosure then the information may be withheld from them.

• Make the referral, if justified, to the appropriate statutory agency with guidance.

From experience, most obstetricians have little knowledge of child protection issues, concentrating instead on the physical progress of the pregnancy. Nevertheless, it would be good practice to communicate any disclosed concerns to them, so that they can care properly and holistically for these women. Obstetricians cannot do this if they have not got a full picture of the woman and her subsequent difficulties and problems. The information will in all probability be a learning curve for them. It would be beneficial for a paediatrician or nurse from the neonatal intensive care unit to become involved antenatally, or at least have knowledge of any pregnant woman caught up with child protection procedures, if the baby is likely to need care in the neonatal intensive care unit once born (for example, a woman with a drug dependency).

You may find having such openness in telling the family about a referral hard to accept and undertake, as you may believe that your actions will be seen as a betrayal of the family. You may feel that any previous good relationship will be undermined or that the family will become hostile towards you. However, honesty is important if the child protection concerns are to be explored thoroughly, and it is important for the family to know that they can trust the professionals and that nothing is being hidden from them. If trust in the professionals is apparent then the family can be involved in any decision-making and planning about their child. This honesty is expected from the professionals dealing with the family and the child (DH, 1995a).

Family members should normally have a right to know what is being said about them and be allowed to contribute to important decisions about their lives and those of their children. It is important to remember that family members know more about their children than any professional can ever know.

Research (DH, 1995b) has endorsed the importance of good relationships between professionals and families in helping to bring about the best possible outcomes for children. However, caution needs to prevail so that partnership with families does not always mean agreeing with the parents, or accepting their version of events for the way forwards, as this may not be in the child's best interests. Not all parents have the ability to safeguard their children even with help and support.

If the baby is born the above procedures remain the same, but in addition a paediatrician will very likely be involved. If the baby shows signs of physical injury that could be non-accidental, then contact with a paediatrician – either community or hospital – with child protection experience will be necessary. If the parents have accessed medical help from their GP, or attended an accident and emergency department and non-accidental injury is suspected, then an automatic referral to an appropriate paediatrician should be made from this contact.

In these circumstances the referral to a statutory agency will, in all probability, be made by someone else. However, your knowledge of the family will be vital and at some stage this knowledge will be ascertained and you will be invited to any meetings and expected to contribute, within the child protection process.

ASSESSING CHILDREN IN NEED

The Department of Health has produced a booklet 'Framework for the Assessment of Children in Need and their Families' which is primarily for use by professionals who are involved in undertaking assessments of children (DH, 2000). In reality this is essentially social workers, within child protection, but it is a useful guide for any professional dealing with child protection procedures and any designated or named health professional for child protection should be well acquainted with it. While social workers have their assessment to make, which is usually lengthy and complex, the assessment framework is a tool in order to integrate with health issues, which are primarily the province of midwives and health visitors. Midwives and health visitors are therefore expected to comply with the assessment framework, which means that all agencies are working towards the same objective. The assessment framework is a systematic way of analysing, understanding and recording what is happening within a family and from this understanding of what are inevitably complex issues and relationships, clear and sound professional judgements can be made.

This assessment framework is designed to be used with other publications and materials for assessing children in need but this particular publication is a cornerstone of quality assessment. A core assessment is defined as an in-depth assessment which addresses the central or most important aspects of the needs of a child and the capacity of his or her parents or caregivers to respond appropriately to these needs within the wider family and community context (DH, 2000).

A child in need can be defined in many different circumstances, for example, a disabled child, a child whose parents die or a child at risk of significant harm from its carers. As this book is about child protection, the focus will be on this latter group of children in need.

Many families seek help from social services and they will all have differing levels of need; many will be helped by advice or practical services or short-term intervention. Some will have complex serious problems that require more detailed assessment, which involve other agencies in the process, leading to appropriate plans and interventions (DH, 2000).

As you will see as this book progresses, the majority of child protection cases that you become involved with will be complex and serious, requiring inter-agency co-operation. In such circumstances the local authority social services department and health organisations have a duty to work together to safeguard and promote the welfare of children in their area who are in need. There is also an expectation that, wherever possible, these children in need are supported so that they can be brought up within their own families by the provision of an appropriate range of services.

If a family has been referred to social services because of concerns about maltreatment and they become recognised as including a child in need then social services are obliged to make enquiries to find out what is happening, and whether further action should be taken in order to protect the child. This obligation is set out under section 47 of the Children Act 1989 (Protection of Children).

The framework used in assessing the degree of intervention in a family in need is illustrated in Figure 3.1. This framework can be found in the DH 2000 publication *Framework for the Assessment*

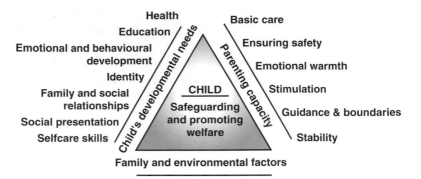

Figure 3.1 The assessment framework (reproduced with permission from DH, 2000).

of Children in Need and their Families and also in 'Working Together'. It is useful to have a working knowledge of this assessment framework, as it will be referred to at inter-agency meetings.

The assessment framework is divided into three areas:

- The developmental needs of the child.
- The capacities of parents or carers to respond to those needs.
- The impact of the wider family and environmental factors on parenting capacity and children.

This assessment framework is represented as a triangle or a pyramid with the child's welfare at its centre. The emphasis is that all assessment activity and subsequent planning and provision of services must focus on ensuring that the child's welfare is safeguarded and promoted.

THE NEXT STAGES OF THE CHILD PROTECTION PROCESS

This can appear complicated but regular involvement with the child protection process will bring with it a familiarity with the procedures. The starting point is the **referral to a statutory agency** following a discussion with your appropriate senior midwife and/or specialist health professionals for child protection. On receipt of this referral by the statutory agency, they must make a decision within 24 hours, which will inform the next stage. The questions that will be posed by this agency will be:

- Does this referral meet their eligibility criteria for being pursued as a child in need?
- Are there concerns about significant harm?
- Has a crime been committed necessitating referral to the police?

If the case does not meet the eligibility criteria for child protection, for instance, a child with a health need, such as living in an inappropriate health environment, this could be re-directed to more appropriate services. If there are concerns about significant harm then the next stage in the child protection process will be undertaken, which would be **background enquiries** and an **initial assessment.** The question that would be posed here by social services would be:

- Do the concerns appear well founded?

This initial assessment by the social services department of all children in need, whether or not there are child protection concerns, should be completed within seven working days from the date of referral. However, if there is reasonable cause to suspect that a child is suffering, or likely to suffer significant harm, this initial assessment may be very brief and enquiries will be made under section 47 (S47) of the Children Act 1989.

The Framework for the Assessment of Children in Need and their Families requests that the initial assessment asks these questions:

- What are the needs of the child and is this a child in need?
- Are the parents able to respond appropriately to the child's needs?
- Is the child being adequately safeguarded from significant harm?
- Are the parents able to promote the child's health and development?
- Is action needed to promote the child's welfare?

In such circumstances, where there are clearly established concerns about significant harm to a child, without co-operation from the parents, which necessitate immediate protection, then S47 enquiries will be pursued. However, it may be obvious at this stage that the parents recognise their difficulties and are willing to co-operate in the best interests of their child. This assessment can then be made under section 17 (S17) of the Children Act 1989. In these circumstances it could mean that more time might be available to make a more thorough assessment.

If, at this stage, following enquiries social services decide to take no further action, feedback will be provided to the referrer. If the referrer was a member of the public this must be done in a manner consistent with respecting the confidentiality of the child and family.

Even when allegations are unsubstantiated, parents and carers can become extremely distressed by the enquiries into their lifestyle. The family can become alarmed, hostile and angry and the midwife may become caught up in the overspill and may need to spend some time soaking up the parents' distress, gently supporting and helping the family to re-establish some equilibrium in their lives.

The background enquiries following a referral about an unborn baby, or new baby, would involve you being asked questions about the family, your involvement and your views. The family health visitor and GP and any other significant professional will also be contacted for information.

In these circumstances, you will be expected to disclose fully any information that you have about the family and the care of their child. Such disclosure is allowed in the public interest and for the initial assessment to have all the known facts available in order to inform the next stage.

This information gathered may result in no further action being taken, other than more appropriate support services being mobilised, or the care may continue under S47 enquiries, or may move into S17 enquiries under the Children Act. If the background enquiries and initial assessment have discovered that the family wish to co-operate with social services in a meaningful way and are actively seeking help, the next step in this process would, in all probability, result in the progression of S17 enquiries and move into a **family support conference.**

A family support conference and subsequent reviews take place within the same timescale as a child protection conference. A family support conference is usual when the concerns are substantiated and the initial assessment of risk has realised that an agreement between the parents and professionals is possible, and that there is meaningful co-operation and agreement regarding the concerns and the way forward. In addition, there are necessary resources available to ensure the safety of the child.

Case history 3.2 gives a good example of section 17 enquiries.

Case history 3.2

Becky and Stuart both have learning disabilities and live independently but within a housing complex with a warden 24 hours a day in case of emergencies. There were serious child protection concerns when Becky became pregnant, regarding their capacity and capability to care for a baby. Both parents realised that they had limitations and they were themselves concerned about what would happen once the baby was born. A strategy meeting was held and the parents attended, along with Stuart's parents. The professionals involved within the strategy discussion realised that Becky and Stuart could not adequately care for their baby, without additional help, and the baby would need to be protected from harm in some way. The police attended the strategy meeting as usual but soon realised that there were no police issues regarding Becky and Stuart.

Stuart's parents were also keen to co-operate with social services to help protect the baby. All members of this family actively knew that they needed help and therefore a family support conference was convened under S17 enquiries.

A package of support was organised for Becky and Stuart when the baby was born. Stuart's parents bought a property for Becky and Stuart to live close to them and these grandparents agreed to care for the baby for parts of every day, and that the baby would sometimes stay overnight with them. This support proved successful and Becky and Stuart managed, with all the help, to care for their baby adequately and lovingly.

If the concerns appear well founded and the child appears to be at risk of significant harm and the case does not fit into support within a family support conference under S17 enquiries, then S47 enquiries will continue. The next stage in this process is a **strategy discussion.**

THE STRATEGY DISCUSSION

A strategy discussion can take place over the telephone, but in reality it is usual for the relevant professionals to meet face to face. The discussion always involves a dialogue between social services and the police. It will also include any other relevant agency that has crucial information about a child. This could be health (for example, a midwife, health visitor, or school nurse) or services such as education or probation. The purpose of this discussion is to agree whether enquiries need to be continued under S47 enquiries and if so to develop a plan of action which will inform the next stage.

A strategy discussion is for professionals only and the parents would not be invited. The strategy discussion will share information between the professionals and will consider:

- Who will be interviewed, by whom, for what purpose and when;
- Who will see the child if the referral is about an older child;
- Any issues arising from disability, race and ethnicity of the child and family;
- The needs of any other child who may be affected;
- What immediate action may be needed to safeguard the child and/or provide interim services and support;
- What information about the strategy discussion will be shared with the family;
- Issues regarding staff safety.

There will be occasions when disclosing information from the strategy meeting to the parents may jeopardise the safety of the child further or harm any police investigation into an alleged offence. In such circumstances the strategy discussion will make very clear details about information to be shared or whether all information will be withheld. For example, a strategy discussion may decide that there are sufficient grounds for removing a baby at birth, but if the parents were in receipt of such information they may disappear or conceal the birth, thus placing the child in serious danger. If the parents were not to be informed, then this would be a joint decision between the professionals involved, and would not be a single agency or single person's decision.

Child protection investigations involve both childcare issues and law enforcement. Close co-operation between social services and the police is therefore essential. The strategy discussion will give a wider view of the family, which will include information from the police of any criminal convictions of either parent or carer. If the initial referral warrants a criminal investigation by the police then they will initiate this.

Any criminal investigation undertaken by the police will proceed concurrently with the child protection process.

If enquiries are to continue, then the next step following the strategy discussion will be carried out according to the plan made at the discussion. It may emerge at any stage that the concerns are not sufficient enough to require the convening of a child protection conference; if so, the enquiries may stop and no further action will be taken or the enquiries may move into S17 enquiries.

The investigation following the strategy discussion will involve interviews with the relevant people, such as the parents, any other significant adults in the child's life and maybe other children living in the household. The question as to who will undertake these interviews will have been decided at the discussion.

If the concerns remain following the investigation then a **child protection conference** will be convened (Figure 3.2).

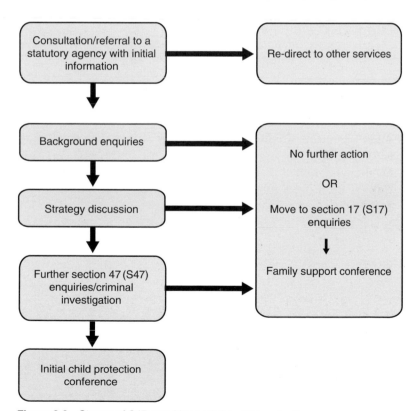

Figure 3.2   Stages of S47 enquiries and the child protection process.

Although section 17 and section 47 refer to sections of the Children Act (1989), the child protection process in Scotland follows the same pathway but does not make reference to these sections of the Act, as they are unique to England and Wales.

Families who understand the child protection process understand the reasons why professionals from the agencies involved need to ask searching and intimate questions. In reality the families, even if treated sensitively and sympathetically, often focus their anger on the workers involved, particularly social workers and the police. This anger can be enhanced if the allegations are unsubstantiated and any correspondence with the family from these agencies must address the distress caused, and whenever possible encourage the families to return to social services when help is needed (DH, 1995a). For some families this may not be enough and long-term counselling may be necessary. It could be helpful for the families to know about self-help groups (see the list of support groups in the appendix).

Midwives are fortunate in that their work brings them into contact with a wide variety of families with varying backgrounds. They can have some escape from families in desperate need that have been caught up in the child protection process. Such needy families can be an emotional drain on a midwife because of the intensity of their emotions and their acute distress, which is highly likely to spill over into anger and hostility, often towards workers who are trying to do their best for the children in difficult circumstances. Life for workers who only ever deal with such families, those who miss out on seeing happy comfortable children being cared for lovingly by their parents, can have additional stresses, which need to be recognised and appreciated by midwives.

ASK YOURSELF

1. Do you know where your local area child protection committee (ACPC) or child protection committee (CPC) policies and procedures are kept?
2. Can you list 10 signs in children that may make you suspect that some form of child abuse is happening?
3. What is the difference between S17 and S47 enquiries under the Children Act 1989?
4. Can you explain the process of child protection enquiries?
5. What agencies are involved with the process?

REFERENCES

Department of Health (DH) (1995a) *The Challenge of Partnership in Child Protection: Practice Guide*. London: The Stationery Office.

Department of Health (DH) (1995b) *Child Protection: Messages from Research*. London: The Stationery Office.

Department of Health (DH) (1997) *Child Protection: Guidance for Senior Nurses, Health Visitors and Midwives and their Managers*. London: The Stationery Office.

Department of Health (DH) (1999) *Working Together to Safeguard Children: A Guide to Inter-agency Working to Safeguard and Promote the Welfare of Children*. London: The Stationery Office.

Department of Health (DH) (2000) *Framework for the Assessment of Children in Need and their Families*. London: The Stationery Office.

Dimond B. (2002) *Legal Aspects of Midwifery*, 2nd edn. Oxford: Books for Midwives Press.

Scottish Office (1998) P*rotecting Children, A Shared Responsibility: Guidance on Inter-agency Co-operation*. Edinburgh: The Stationery Office.

FURTHER READING

Chapman T. (2002) Safeguarding the welfare of children: 1. *British Journal of Midwifery*, 10(9):569–572.

Cochrane Review (update 1998) Home-based social support for socially disadvantaged mothers. Oxford: Cochrane Library.

Department of Health (DH) (1989) *An Introduction to the Children Act 1989*. London: The Stationery Office.

Department of Health (DH) (2002) S*afeguarding Children in Whom Illness is Fabricated or Induced*. London: DH Publications (or available from the website *www.doh.gov.uk/acpc*).

Howe D., Brandon M., Hinings D, Schofield G. (1999) *Attachment Theory, Child Maltreatment and Family Support*. London: Macmillan.

Klaus M., Kennell M, Klaus P. (1995) *Bonding*. London: Mandarin Paperbacks.

Scottish Office (1995) *Scotland's Children: A Brief Guide to the Children (Scotland) Act 1995*. Edinburgh: The Stationery Office.

Stower S. (2000) The principles and practice of child protection, *Nursing Standard*, 14(17):48–55.

4

The child protection conference

The most important person at a child protection conference is the child, whether born or unborn, and this must be focused on at all times. The child protection conference enables the professionals involved with the family to meet together to assess all the relevant information pertinent to the family, to plan how to safeguard the child and consequently promote his welfare.

Midwives often find attending a child protection conference daunting and you will need some support if asked to attend. Someone with more experience than yourself should attend the conference with you, such as the named midwife in child protection, a midwife with the relevant expertise and knowledge or your manager. You need to familiarise yourself with the procedure for a child protection conference beforehand so that you are not caught off guard, as the conference is a formal occasion with a set agenda. There will be a variety of other professionals attending as the conference has multi-agency representation. Those professionals who are invited to attend are required to give their professional judgement and some analysis of risk to the child's future safety, health and development.

The conference is a forum for bringing together the family with the relevant professionals engaged in the child protection procedures for the particular family. It provides an opportunity to pool and exchange all the information available, to plan together the action necessary to protect the child from harm.

A conference can only be convened by an agency with statutory powers to do so; these are the social services or the NSPCC. A conference will follow a referral, from whatever source, provided that the processes following the referral lead to a suspicion that the child is suffering from or likely to suffer from significant harm. This detailed gathering of information and initial assessment under section 47 (S47) enquiries are discussed in detail in Chapter 3.

The first child protection conference convened on an unborn or new baby is called an **initial child protection conference** and will be held within 15 working days of the strategy meeting. Any conference convened following the initial child protection conference is known as a **review child protection conference** and this must be held within 3 months of the initial child protection conference and thereafter, if needed, at a maximum of 6-monthly intervals. If an initial child protection conference is convened once the baby is born it is highly unlikely that you will be invited to the review conference, as your involvement with the family will have ceased long before.

MEMBERS INVITED TO A CHILD PROTECTION CONFERENCE

Social services are the key agency when child protection matters are dealt with and they invite the differing agencies to a child protection conference. The attendance of the main social worker assigned to the family is obviously vital; this social worker may be a senior practitioner, which in essence is a senior social worker who has influence and expertise within child protection. Agencies always invited to a child protection conference are health disciplines and the police. The police normally have specialist officers who deal with child protection issues and have received specialist training in this area. Most cities have a separate police department that deals exclusively with child protection, which ensures that the officers dealing with this work have the skills and knowledge that are necessary for the child protection procedures to run smoothly.

The health disciplines that are invited to a child protection conference, according to the age of the child, are: the family GP, the family's health visitor, midwives (both hospital and community-based if a baby is involved), school nurses and paediatric nurses. In the case of a baby it would be unusual for a school nurse to be invited unless there were other school-age children in the family and their input was relevant to the safety of the new baby. In general any child protection conference that a midwife attends would usually involve the presence of the family health visitor; often this is the only other health discipline involved, as it is unusual for GPs to attend a child protection conference, but they are always invited.

Other agencies invited by social services to a child protection conference, according to the circumstances, are: probation officers, teachers, educational welfare officers, foster parents, the local authority solicitor, a children's guardian (formerly known as guardian *ad litem)*, the NSPCC or any other relevant professional who has had contact with the family. There may also be representation from other voluntary agencies (although this is generally for older children), such as NCH, which is a leading children's charity committed to supporting children and young people by providing them with opportunities to reach their full potential.

Child protection conferences can therefore be large and involve many people. An example of a particularly small conference is illustrated in Case history 4.1.

Case history 4.1

A conference is held about Samantha and Jack, the parents of a 2-week-old baby. The conference was convened because Samantha had her first baby while still a teenager and this baby had to be removed into care as the baby was neglected. The circumstances at the time led to the baby remaining in care and subsequently being adopted. This child was born 7 years earlier. While pregnant this time Samantha had some supportive social work involvement and it was clear that she had matured greatly since the birth of her first child, and she and Jack appeared to be caring and committed would-be parents. A decision was therefore made that a pre-birth child protection conference was not necessary but this conference in question would be held once the baby was born, to assess the parenting abilities of the couple with the new baby.

The invited members at this conference were the allocated social worker, the health visitor, the midwife and the trust's named midwife for child protection. Both parents attended, making only eight people altogether. The professionals in attendance were: the chair, the minute taker, the allocated social worker, health visitor, midwife and named midwife. The police chose not to attend because there were no police charges against either of the parents and no concerns regarding this new baby.

The family's social worker gave a positive report about the family and felt that the baby was well cared for, appropriately handled and that positive parenting skills were readily apparent. The midwife had a similar report and stated that Samantha had attended all her antenatal care, had been committed to preparing for the baby and Samantha and Jack together shared the care of this baby and that the care was loving and consistent.

A unanimous decision was made that the baby should not be registered on the child protection register and after discussion with the family, Samantha and Jack felt that they wanted to manage on their own, without any further outside support, as they felt that they were capable and good enough parents. It was impressed on Samantha and Jack that if they felt that they were beginning to find caring for their baby difficult then they must access help quickly. This they agreed to do.

This was a straightforward conference and all parties left the conference happy, as it was evident that no further action needed to be taken.

In contrast, a child protection conference for Case history 4.2 heralded the presence of 12 different professionals. The parents attended the conference as well, therefore this conference consisted of 14 people including the minute taker. This is obviously a large conference for a complicated family. The professionals at this conference consisted of the chair of conference, two social workers because of the complexity of the case and a team manager from social services, the health visitor and her team leader for support, a community midwife and the named midwife in child protection for support, two police officers, a probation officer and the local authority solicitor.

Case history 4.2

Gemma and Gary both had a difficult history. Gemma had a 2-year-old daughter that had been removed from her care and lived with her maternal grandmother. Gemma had given her own lifestyle priority over that of her new baby. She would go out to clubs and pubs and leave her daughter unattended in the house. The police were called several times by neighbours but Gemma continued her chosen lifestyle. Gemma saw her daughter at specified times twice a week. Gemma was content with this and did not want to gain custody of her daughter.

Gary was a travelling salesman and spent most of his time on the road. Gemma would regularly accompany him even at the detriment of her own health while pregnant. Gemma would default an antenatal visit if Gary wanted her with him. Gemma did not know where she would give birth, she would say that she would go to whichever was the nearest hospital on her travels with Gary. However, Gemma had not found out the telephone numbers of any hospitals on Gary's route, which was obviously of great concern.

Gary had several convictions for the rape of teenage girls; one was his own stepdaughter whom he regularly 'groomed' for the occasions. Gary received a custodial sentence and while in prison became friends with another schedule 1 offender called Brian.

Gary was released from prison and moved back into the home he shared with Gemma. Gemma was thrilled to have him back. When Brian was released, several weeks later, he was homeless and Gary invited him to live with them also.

This was a long and protracted conference, which was necessary to enable everyone to have a contribution enabling the safest outcome for the baby. Gemma and Gary considered themselves to be able parents and were regularly hostile to the professionals during the conference.

A decision was made to register the baby on the child protection register under the category of likelihood of sexual abuse. The local authority solicitor informed the conference that the criteria were met in order to go to court once the baby was born to apply for an interim care order. It was felt by the conference members that it was unsafe for the baby to return home with Gemma and Gary, once the baby was born, and that a foster placement would need to be found to keep the baby safe.

> **Case History 4.2—cont'd**
>
> A national alert was sent out to all maternity units with these details should the baby be born elsewhere.
> The baby was actually born within its own area and an interim care order (ICO) was granted by the court on the day that the baby was born, granting the local authority parental responsibility for the child. Gemma and Gary were encouraged to care for their baby in the unit but went home without the baby and the baby went into foster care with regular visits from Gemma and Gary. The baby was subsequently placed for adoption, as Gemma and Gary gradually lost interest in their baby and stopped visiting him.

The parents (or those with parental responsibility) are always invited to a child protection conference. It is only in extreme circumstances that they are not, for example, if there were a real threat of physical violence from a parent or if the child would be placed in further danger by the involvement of the parents. The decision not to invite a parent to a child protection conference is never taken lightly and the decision has to be justified thoroughly. In the case of a parent being excluded on the grounds of potential violence they will receive the minutes of the conference in order to be kept informed of the decisions being made by the professionals. If the parents are excluded, because the child could be placed in further danger by their involvement, then a decision may be made not to inform the parents of the conference or the contents within it. An example of this may be in the case of a child where the parents are fabricating or inducing an illness in their child (factitious illness by proxy, previously known as Munchausen's syndrome by proxy) or some cases of sexual abuse.

OBSERVERS

The parents or parent may choose to be accompanied to the conference by a friend, family member or supporter to offset some of their feelings of apprehension. This supporter cannot be a member of the conference and is not allowed to contribute to the discussion taking place. The parents will know this in advance and it would be re-iterated by the chair of conference at the start of discussions. Parents can invite their solicitor as their supporter, the role though remains the same as above and the solicitor cannot join in the discussion taking place, or make any suggestions or decision on behalf of their client. The advantage of the parents taking their solicitor is that any facts not understood by the parents can be explained by their solicitor later. The solicitor is allowed to make notes and the advantage to them is that they have access to the information from conference at first hand, and can therefore support their clients more appropriately at a later date.

There may be other observers at a conference; for instance, a student midwife, student health visitor or indeed any qualified professional who needs to learn about child protection procedures and needs to see how the procedures actually operate. It is a fruitful way of learning. However, no one can be taken to a conference without first seeking permission from the chair. The chair has the overall responsibility for deciding who may or may not attend a particular conference. Observers cannot join the discussion or decide whether a baby should be registered on the child protection register.

CHAIR OF CONFERENCE

An independent chairperson, who has received training to undertake this task, chairs all child protection conferences. Most independent chairs are qualified social workers who have worked in a senior capacity within child protection. The chair is completely independent of any work, operational or line management responsibilities that have taken place for this family. The independent chair therefore has a completely objective overall view of the family that will emerge from the conference. The chair can undertake more than one child protection conference with a particular family, for instance, chairing the initial conference and also the review conference(s).

However good the preparation has been beforehand in preparing for conference, the chairperson remains vital to a positive outcome.

The chair has the power to exclude any member if there is a risk of violence and if the evidence suggests that the conference will be disrupted. This will be in exceptional circumstances only and the justifiable reasons for the exclusion will be documented in the minutes. The excluded member will still be encouraged, probably through their social worker or solicitor, to communicate their views to the conference and this input is necessary to gain a full picture to make the best possible decision for the child. The communication could be in the form of a letter from the family, should the family not wish to have their views expressed through another person. Most independent chairs would offer, if possible, to meet the parents before the conference, even if they are not allowed into the conference, to establish their views if no other way of communication had been ascertained.

The chair of the conference is crucial in implementing the smooth running of the conference. The chairperson's role is expected to establish fairness, openness and honesty in which the family and professionals work together for the benefit of the child. The chair will meet with the parents in a separate room to the professionals before the conference, this will possibly be in the room that the conference will be held in, so that the parents can familiarise themselves with the room before the entry of the other members of conference. The chair will explain the process to the parents and try and relax them if at all possible. This meeting is also to try and make sure that the parents understand the purpose and decision-making processes that will be undertaken by the conference. The chair will then take the parents into the room (if they are not already in it) which is to be used for conference. Following this the chair will gather the waiting professionals and invite them into the room already occupied by the parents.

The conference is usually held round a conference table. The agenda for the conference will be laid out for everyone to see and water and tissues are usually to hand as well. The first time you walk into the room for a conference it will feel daunting, as you will not know what to expect and the family will be familiar to you, and you may feel awkward in their presence. You may have only seen this family in your antenatal clinic, or on a hospital ward, and so the unfamiliar place with so many other professionals around you may feel confusing. Just imagine – if you feel like this how must it feel for the parents? The reason that the chair will make sure that the parents are in the room first is to try and offset some of those feelings for them, by them not having to walk into a room already full of professionals, most of whom will have had some contact in one way or another with the family. However nervous you feel, they will be feeling much worse. The chair of conference will try and enable this process to be as smooth as possible.

The chair is responsible for ensuring that the conference is conducted in an anti-discriminatory manner, ensuring that everyone uses unambiguous language. You need to remember that words which are familiar within our profession may make little sense to the parents or to the professionals from other disciplines and agencies. Likewise the chair should ensure that you understand any aspects of others agencies' reports that will be unfamiliar to you. The chair needs to consider at all times any disabilities or cultural differences that need to be taken into consideration and accounted for when making decisions or developing plans.

The chair will encourage straightforward discussion and will be responsible for ensuring that the process or discussions taking place do not overwhelm the parents.

As you can imagine, even the most straightforward conference will take some time, an hour at least. A more complex case can take several hours. It is important to arrive at conference at least 20 minutes before the start, as you will need to read the social worker's report, which will be available to you in the waiting room, before the commencement of the conference.

OUTLINE AGENDA FOR AN INITIAL CHILD PROTECTION CONFERENCE

A conference can be held anywhere, provided that the room is private, it does not have to be on social services premises.

It is always wise to arrive early for a conference, as the time given to you is the time of starting. However, normally the (main) social worker's report will be available for you to read on arrival while waiting for conference to start. You will therefore need to give yourself some time to read this report, which can be lengthy according to the circumstances.

Once you are taken into the conference room and seated you will possibly see other members writing their names and agency on a specific card, and some marker pens are available for use. This is useful for you to know who the other members are and what agency they represent. You do not need to write much, just your name and midwife is quite sufficient.

The following agenda will give you an idea of the format; however, some adaptation may take place from this outline.

1. The purpose and process of the conference will be explained by the chair.

2. An equal opportunities statement including confidentiality and the use of third party information.

3. Introductions and apologies.

4. The social worker whose report you will have read while waiting will present the report to conference by picking out and highlighting the main points. Usually at the end of the report the parents' comments are documented as to their view of the report. The report will have been thoroughly shared with them in the days or weeks leading up to conference to make sure that they have had time to digest the information being presented and to allow for any misunderstandings they may have.

5. Agency reports. You will be expected to write a report for conference. It is always good practice to share your report with the family beforehand so that there are no surprises for them. If you have little experience of child protection it is advisable to do this only if you have discussed the issues with someone else in advance. Families can react in different ways to reports and you must not put yourself on the receiving end of verbal aggression unnecessarily. The chair will decide which order the reports will take and will try and make the reports sequential. It is usual for the main social worker to outline the current situation first, referring to her report as necessary. She will outline the current situation, the reasons for the referral and an explanation of why the conference is being held. At a conference for an unborn baby or new baby then it is possible that you may be asked to speak next and the first professional to speak after the social worker's report.

6. Other relevant information. Questions or comments from the invited members of conference or clarifications are sought. At this point any third party information that is necessary for the safety of the child may be shared. The parents and any family supporters will be asked to leave at this point and they will be taken to another room to wait while the relevant information is shared. For example, at Gemma and Gary's conference they were asked to leave when details about Brian and his schedule 1 status were taken into consideration, because he was living in the same house, and intended staying long term even after the baby had been born. This information is highly relevant to the members of conference and they must have the information on a 'need to know' basis. The police will give out relevant information and any convictions would need to be taken into account by conference. As the information is about a third party

the parents, and any supporter that they may have, cannot be present for this information. Once this information has been discussed during this part of the conference, the parents will then be invited back into the room. The chair should know in advance about any potential third party information that needs to be disclosed. This is necessary in order for the chair to make sure that the parents understand what will happen in advance, that they will be asked to leave the conference, when this information is being imparted.

7. Legal advice from the local authority solicitor, if present, may be sought following the agency reports. This would be to ascertain whether proceedings should be issued through the courts if necessary. If the parents are still in the room because there was no relevant third party information then they will be asked to leave while the legal advice is being given.

8. The chair will summarise the key points to assist the conference in undertaking an assessment of risk.

9. The assessment of risk will be given careful consideration and the risks and protective factors concerning the child will be analysed separately by conference members.

10. A decision will be made by the invited professional conference members on whether to register the child on the child protection register. Each invited professional in turn will be asked their thoughts on registration and their decision. There will usually be some documentation before you at the conference giving an explanation of the criteria for registration and the professionals present need to decide whether those criteria have been met. The question to always ask yourself when considering registering a child is: *Is this child at continuing risk of significant harm?*

11. The date of the review child protection conference if the child is registered.

RECOGNITION OF SIGNIFICANT HARM

It is very difficult to quantify exactly what constitutes significant harm but the following list may give you some guide:

- Any allegation of sexual abuse.
- Parents who may present a high risk to children because of:
  (i) domestic violence

(ii) drug and alcohol abuse

(iii) mental health problems.

- Physical injury caused by assault or neglect which requires medical attention, especially any injury to a baby under the age of 1 year.
- Repeated incidents of physical harm that are unlikely to constitute significant harm in themselves but collectively may do so.
- Contact with a person assessed as presenting a risk to children.
- Children who live in a low warmth, high criticism environment which is likely to have an adverse impact on their emotional development.
- Children who suffer from persistent neglect.
- Children living in a household where there is domestic violence likely to lead to physical or emotional harm.
- A child living in a household or having significant contact with a schedule 1 offender.
- Children who may be involved in prostitution (DH, 2000b).
- Other circumstances where professional judgement and/or evidence suggests that a child's health, development or welfare may be significantly harmed. (Norfolk ACPC, 2000)

FEMALE GENITAL MUTILATION

Female genital mutilation (circumcision) is illegal unless there are specific medical grounds for its performance. Other than health grounds, undertaking this procedure on a child is likely to be, or has been, subject to significant harm taking place.

SCHEDULE 1 OFFENDER

A schedule 1 offender is someone who has been convicted of any offence against a child, which is listed in schedule 1 of the Children and Young Persons Act 1933 or schedule 1 of the Criminal Procedure (Scotland) Act 1995. A child protection conference, except in exceptional circumstances, would always be convened if a schedule 1 offender began living with children, if they were to become a parent or started to have significant contact with a particular child or children. Anyone convicted of such an offence resulting in becoming a schedule 1 offender would always be notified to social services.

WRITING YOUR REPORT FOR A CHILD PROTECTION CONFERENCE

There is an expectation that every agency attending a child protection conference will submit a report regarding their involvement with the family. This is not expected to be particularly lengthy. The social worker's report, based on the assessment framework, is expected to be comprehensive and should give all the background details of the family; your report should be much more to the point. Your report should be typed, factual and checked for accuracy. It is always helpful to explain any words that are unfamiliar outside our profession. Whoever is supporting you at conference will help and advise in your preparation of the report. This report will be collected at conference along with everyone else's and retained on file in case the information is needed at a later stage.

If you know that you have a family that is involved in the child protection procedures, it is useful to make explicit contemporaneous records every time you have contact with them, at any stage of their pregnancy. Dates and times are usually significant and these notes will make writing your report much easier.

It is helpful to have the information from your report in front of you at conference as it will be an aide-mémoire and will give you confidence when speaking. You may prefer to read your report to conference to give the other members the picture that you are presenting. If in doubt ask the chair, when it is your turn to speak, which way they would prefer you to give your information.

Your report must give a balanced view of the family. It is imperative that you keep to facts only and not be side-tracked by opinion in your report. For example, it would be unacceptable to write such comments as 'this is a very dirty house and Jane cannot possibly bring up a baby with so much dirt and mess around'. This is clearly an opinion and must be avoided. A factual summary would be expected such as 'Jane finds keeping the house clean and tidy quite difficult and the house is often dirty and messy'. Your comments must stop at this point as you would not be expected to give an opinion on whether the baby should remain in the house or not. This sharing of information is one of the purposes of the conference, and then decisions are made collectively as to the future welfare of the child.

THROUGH THE MIDWIFE'S EYES

Midwives usually find a child protection conference daunting because the nature of the work is very different from everyday practice. While most midwives have contact with families going through the rigours of the child protection proceedings, it does not form the main thrust of most midwives' work. Routinely a midwife is working with families who are happy to welcome children into their lives and who bring up their children with success, mutual love and enjoyment. They are pleased with their children and glow with pride when they talk about them. They bond with their babies and the babies in turn have secure attachments to their mothers.

It can therefore be difficult for midwives when they are catapulted out of their usual daily work. Midwives often become distressed when the details of a family are discussed openly at conference and the midwife may find herself in an unfamiliar world, where child abuse has taken place, where criminal convictions of the parents are disclosed, where older children have been profoundly affected by the physical or emotional abuse that they have suffered, where children have been removed from their parents. Prostitution, drugs and pornography can all be involved; it is unfamiliar and upsetting; be prepared to feel uncomfortable about information that may be relayed.

Your contribution at conference is of worth and will be noted. It will be valued, separate from, but networked in with, the other agencies that are involved. Different agencies may not agree with each other's view but by co-operating together the best possible outcome for the child's welfare should be secured. You may feel overwhelmed by the intensity and the vast amount of information that other agencies have about the family. You have to remember that other agencies, for example, social services, probation and teachers may have a history with the family spanning many years and not just the few months that midwives are involved with families. It is helpful to remember though that the time that midwives are involved with a family is a time of particular change and stress, and the information imparted about the family under these circumstances is highly significant and relevant.

'Working Together' has this to say about a pre-birth conference:

Where S47 enquiries give rise to concern that an unborn child may be at future risk of significant harm, the social services department may need to convene an initial child protection conference prior to the child's birth. Such a conference should have the same status, and proceed in the same way, as other initial child protection conferences, including decisions about registration. The involvement of midwifery services is vital in such cases.

Midwives must always remember that if an unborn baby is registered on the child protection register, then it is vital that communication channels are put in place so that the key social worker is informed of the birth as soon as possible. It is imperative that someone takes responsibility for this task. According to the circumstances the key social worker may need to put immediate safeguards in place to protect the new baby. This cannot be done in advance, as an unborn baby has no rights or status in law. The child only acquires these rights once he is born and has taken his first breath. An application can then be made to the courts if this is what is planned. You will be asked the sex of the baby and it is usual for the baby's name to be requested prior to the application to court.

Because of the fact that midwives work in an intimate way with families they can develop an insight into the family that others may not have seen. You may have a unique view of the family and, according to this view, different emotions will be heightened within you. You may feel that compared with other families these particular parents are inadequate and the baby would be better off elsewhere; you can see nothing positive about the family at all. There is a possibility that the family may have been hostile to you at some point and this may also cloud your judgement. In these circumstances it could annoy you that members of the conference are trying to give a balanced view of the family by drawing out the positive comments about them, or finding areas of worth that could be expanded, as well as bringing out the concerns which brought the family to conference in the first place.

Conversely you may feel that this family has struggled against the odds to cope, that you have supported the family and that the family should not have to endure the added stress of the child protection procedures. By becoming familiar with the child protection procedures it may be easier to stand back and be more objective, acknowledging the most important factor of the conference, that of exploring the future well-being of the unborn baby or baby.

Emotions from the family can be high during a conference; they may feel got at, unsupported, frightened and angry. Tensions may spill over, tears may flow, and one or both of them may walk out.

This could concern you and you may feel that other members of conference are not reacting appropriately towards the expressed emotions. It is essential to remain calm and not rush over to 'help' the family. The chair will cope with any interruptions or difficulties; they are not for you to deal with.

The acute emotions felt by the family will resolve. You may be shocked that some families can be manipulative and will endeavour to play the professionals off against each other. This may be a situation that you have not found yourself in before. However, you need to make sure that you don't get influenced by the family, as the agencies more used to conferences will have experienced such scenarios many times, and will have no hesitation in informing conference of what the family may be saying about them or other conference members.

Following the conference it is important that you seek out an appropriate colleague and spend some time de-briefing. It is important to do this so that you are not left carrying 'emotional luggage' that does not belong to you. If there is something that you have not understood, and did not ask for clarification at conference, then it is perfectly appropriate to seek an explanation from the chair afterwards.

DECISION-MAKING

Conference members (not observers) will make a decision as to whether the child should be placed on the **child protection register**. Each member will be asked for his or her views by the chair of conference. It is always helpful to give some reasoning to your view when asked about registration. If you have not attended a conference before, or feel more inhibited than other members, then make sure that the chair is aware of this; they will then take this into consideration when commencing asking conference members for their views on registration.

To place a child on the child protection register the test is:

1. The child can be shown to have suffered ill treatment or impairment of health or development as a result of physical, emotional or sexual abuse or neglect *and* professional judgement is that further ill treatment or impairment is likely **or**
2. Professional judgement, substantiated by the findings of enquiries in this individual case or by research evidence, is that

the child is likely to suffer ill treatment or the impairment of health and development as a result of physical, emotional, sexual abuse or neglect.

If you have not been to a child protection conference it is worth telling the chair when you introduce yourself at the beginning of conference. The chair will then be sensitive to this when asking about registration of the child and may ask others, more used to the proceedings, to speak first. If you are not sure how to respond to the process then it is acceptable to seek such clarification from the chair.

The child may be registered under one or more of the following categories: emotional harm, physical harm, sexual abuse or neglect. Each member will give a view as to which category the child should be registered under; however, the chair will have the final say on this aspect.

If the decision has been made to register a child then the conference will have to make some decisions on ongoing care. The conference will identify a named **key worker** (from social services), identify a **core group** and formulate a **child protection plan**.

Any child placed on the child protection register must have a **core assessment** according to the *Framework for the Assessment of Children in Need and their Families* (DH, 2000a) completed by the social services department in partnership with the appropriate agencies. Appropriate agencies would be according to the age of a child; a midwife would be appropriate for the core group and involvement with the core assessment if the conference were on an unborn baby. The midwife would be expected to assess the parents' parenting capacity; for example, their interactions with the baby, everyday caregiving and to some extent the parents' behaviour and interaction with each other.

CONFIDENTIALITY

The NMC (2002) document 'Code of professional conduct' says this about confidentiality: 'As a registered nurse or midwife, you must protect confidential information' (p. 7). The document is explicit about treating information about patients and clients as confidential and that the information should only be used for the purposes for which it was given. The text continues that it is impractical to obtain consent every time you need to share information with others and that you should ensure that patients and clients understand that some information may be made available to other members of the team involved in the delivery of care.

Paragraph 5.3 (NMC, 2002) says:

If you are required to disclose information outside the team that will have personal consequences for patients or clients, you must obtain their consent. If the patient or client withholds consent, or if consent cannot be obtained for whatever reason, disclosures may be made only where:

- They can be justified in the public interest (usually where disclosure is essential to protect the patient or client or someone else from the risk of significant harm).
- They are required by law or by order of a court.

Child protection is about protecting children from the risk of significant harm; therefore in these circumstances it is appropriate for you to disclose information to other agencies outside your own team, even without consent from the parents.

Dimond (1994) also says that a breach of confidentiality is justified in the public interest if there is any suspicion of child abuse. Such information should be passed on to the appropriate agencies without fear of a successful action for breach of confidentiality by the parents. In Dimond (2002) she says that midwives should ensure that they only disclose confidential information on the justification of the public interest if they can explain and record why the public interest arises; some of these circumstances are detailed as follows:

- A concern that a client was harming her existing child(ren).
- A concern that a client may harm her baby when born.
- A concern that the client may harm herself.

It is obviously the first two situations that would precipitate the initiation of any child protection procedures.

Paragraph 5.4 (NMC, 2002) says: 'Where there is an issue of child protection, you must act at all times in accordance with national and local policies'. Your local policy will probably tell you to speak to a senior colleague with knowledge of child protection if you are concerned about a family. Any interchange between you and a senior colleague would be a legitimate interchange and would not be breaching confidentiality.

By the time you reach the point of a child protection conference you are therefore divulging information on a 'need to know' basis because of the exceptional circumstances in order to protect a child from harm. However, it is imperative that you remember the purposes of the 'need to know' information that is being divulged to others and that this does not give you freedom to discuss the issues freely outside of conference, other than with those team members involved in the immediate delivery of care.

THE CHILD PROTECTION PLAN

The child protection plan is a detailed plan of actions instigated at the initial child protection conference. The needs of the child and parents will be expressed and the plan will consist of any work that needs to be undertaken with the family, including any monitoring of the family or request for any specialist examination, for instance, from a psychologist. The plan is a tool to monitor the way forward for the family and the progress that is being made. The key worker nominated at conference will co-ordinate and facilitate this child protection plan. The core group chosen will be a small group working together who will work closely with the family and meet at intervals to share information. Although the key worker has the lead role there is an expectation that all members of the core group are jointly responsible for the formation and implementation of the child protection plan, refining as necessary and monitoring the progress against specified objectives. A midwife is usually recommended to be a part of this core group if the baby is unborn. It is unlikely that a midwife would be involved if the baby had already been born.

The initial child protection conference is responsible for agreeing an outline child protection plan and the professionals and parents should develop the finer details of the plan within the core group. The aim of the plan is to:

• Safeguard the child from further harm.
• Promote the child's health and development.
• Provided that it is in the best interest of the child, to support the family and the wider family members to promote the welfare of the child, preferably within the child's own home.

The core group will meet at intervals to pool their information and to make sure that there is a continued focus on the plan of actions and adherence to the child protection plan. The parents are also invited to core group meetings. It is vital that this group communicates effectively as it is the pivot of the ongoing future and outcome for this family. The overall findings of the core group will be fed into the next child protection conference, which will be a review conference, the date of which will have been set at the initial conference and will be held within 3 months of the initial conference.

A WRITTEN AGREEMENT

'Working Together' says:

Parents should be clear about the causes of concern which resulted in the child's name being placed on the child protection register, what needs to change, and about what is expected of them as part of the plan for safeguarding the child. All parties should be clear about the respective roles and responsibilities of family members and different agencies in implementing the plan. It is good practice to produce a written agreement as part of, or additional to the plan, which is negotiated between the child, the family and professionals regarding the implementation of the plan. (p. 59)

CONFERENCE RECORDS

Minutes will be taken by someone whose sole task is to take the conference minutes, which are then circulated as speedily as possible following the conference. In reality a synopsis and the child protection plan may be circulated quickly but the full conference minutes may take several weeks to be received. The minutes will be circulated to all the invited members of conference including the parents, but only provided that they have legal parental authority (legal parental authority is discussed in detail in Chapter 8). Any excluded parent or a parent who chose not to attend will also get a copy. The minutes are strictly private and confidential for obvious reasons and must be kept in a safe place. These minutes cannot be shown to anyone without the permission of conference.

ASK YOURSELF

1. What is the purpose of a child protection conference?
2. Who is invited to a child protection conference?
3. What is contained in the agenda for the child protection conference?
4. What is the role of the key social worker?
5. Who is involved within the core group?
6. What is the purpose of the child protection plan?

REFERENCES

Department of Health (DH) (1999) *Working Together to Safeguard Children: A Guide to Inter-agency Working to Safeguard and Promote the Welfare of Children.* London: The Stationery Office.

Department of Health (DH) (2000a) *Framework for the Assessment of Children in Need and their Families.* London: The Stationery Office.

Department of Health (DH) (2000b) *Safeguarding Children Involved in Prostitution: Supplementary Guidance to Working Together to Safeguard Children.* London: DH Publications.

Dimond B. (1994) *Legal Aspects of Midwifery,* 1st edn. Oxford: Books for Midwives Press.

Dimond B. (2002) *Legal Aspects of Midwifery,* 2nd edn. Oxford: Books for Midwives Press.

Norfolk Area Child Protection Committee (2000) *A Guide to Inter-Agency Working to Safeguard and Promote the Welfare of Children.* Norfolk ACPC.

Nursing & Midwifery Council (NMC) (2002) *Code of Professional Conduct.* London: NMC.

Scottish Office (1998) *Protecting Children, A Shared Responsibility: Guidance on Inter-agency Co-operation.* Edinburgh: The Stationery Office.

FURTHER READING

Department of Health (DH) (2002) *Safeguarding Children in Whom Illness is Fabricated or Induced.* London: DH Publications (or available from the website *www.doh.gov.uk/acpc*).

Fraser J. (1994) Protecting the child. *Nursing Times,* 90(48):54–56.

Miller S. (2002) Child abuse and domestic violence. *British Journal of Midwifery,* 10(9):565–568.

Price S., Baird K. (2003) Tackling domestic violence: an audit of professional practice. *The Practising Midwife,* 6(3):15–18.

Scott L. (2002) Child protection: the role of communication. *Nursing Times,* 98(18):34–36.

5

The child protection register

The child protection register is a list of names of children who are considered to be at a continuing risk of suffering significant harm and are in need of active safeguarding. A child or unborn baby is entered onto the register following an initial child protection conference. The child protection register is strictly controlled by a custodian of the register and can only be accessed by specified personnel from all the agencies involved with child protection.

While the previous chapter addressed the legal status of an unborn baby, in explaining why a court order cannot be secured on a child until it is born, nevertheless an unborn baby can be pencilled onto the child protection register and formally entered once born. The categories for consideration of registration are the same as a child once born.

If asked, midwives often assume that the child protection register is kept in the accident and emergency department, and imagine it to be like our delivery register where different disciplines of staff browse through it from time to time, without anyone as much as raising an eyebrow. Nothing could be further from the truth and the social services department for your particular area will be responsible for the management and maintenance of the register. The care of the register conforms to recommendations from the Department of Health and each social services department throughout the country is accountable for its own register.

The custody of the register is carefully controlled and someone is charged with this task. In England and Wales this is someone usually known as the custodian of the child protection register and in Scotland the keeper of the register. You may find it of interest to find out who is the custodian or keeper of your local child protection register.

The register is a confidential computerised record of the relevant children and it also keeps a record of any siblings of the child, and the name of the abusing adult. This is important as the adult may move to another family and could therefore pose a risk to a different set of children, and this would trigger off a separate child protection investigation to ensure the safety of the children within the new home. In addition to this, a record is kept of any enquiries requesting knowledge about a child, as to whether or not they are on the register. It is usual practice to make a formal child protection referral, once a certain number of enquiries are made about a particular child. The register is designed to be a tool, to make the relevant professionals aware of any children in their area that may be in need of protection.

If a child moves away from the area it is the duty of the custodian to formally notify the details to the relevant custodian in the new area.

Once a child's name has been placed on the register the **core group** must meet within 10 working days of the initial child protection conference. The aim of the core group is to be jointly responsible for implementing the **child protection plan**.

CRITERIA FOR CHILD PROTECTION REGISTRATION

If the child protection conference decides that the child is at continuing risk of significant harm then his or her name will be placed on the child protection register.

The test is that either:

• The child can be shown to have suffered ill treatment or impairment of health or development as a result of physical, emotional or sexual abuse or neglect, *and* professional judgement is that further ill treatment or impairment is likely or

• Professional judgement, substantiated by the findings of enquiries in this individual case or by research evidence, is that the child is likely to suffer ill treatment or the impairment of health and development as a result of physical, emotional, sexual abuse or neglect.

If the initial conference has been convened on an unborn baby then it is difficult to place the unborn baby in the former category, as it could be very difficult to show that the child has already suffered harm; the projected professional judgement would need to be considered.

THE CHILD PROTECTION PLAN

The aim of the plan is to:

- Safeguard the child from future harm.
- Promote the child's health and development.
- Support the family to promote the welfare of their child provided that it is in the best interests of the child.
- Plan the work to be carried out in order to achieve de-registration.

Case history 5.1 is an excellent example of agencies working effectively together, thus ensuring the safety of a baby, both before it was born and afterwards, by the provision of a robust child protection plan. It is hard to imagine what the consequences may have been for Lily and Chloe had it not been for the initiation of the child protection procedures and the child protection plan set up to safeguard Lily.

Case history 5.1

A child protection conference was held on the unborn baby of Chloe. Chloe was studying at university and became pregnant while home for the summer in a quiet seaside resort. The father, Colm, lived locally and Chloe knew him from school. They had an exciting but short-lived affair together. Colm had a history of mental illness and had been sectioned under the Mental Health Act several times. He abused amphetamines and alcohol and had convictions for common assault and criminal damage.

Chloe ended the affair when Colm started treating her violently. Chloe was admitted to the delivery suite several times in her pregnancy with bruises to her stomach; Colm regularly abused her and consequently the unborn baby was in danger because of his violence. Once Chloe stated her intention of leaving Colm he threatened to commit suicide or kill her. Several times Chloe felt that she could not leave her house as Colm would become unreasonably possessive and jealous and demand to know where she was at all times of the day. A child protection conference was subsequently convened following a referral to social services from the midwives on the delivery suite when Chloe began telling her story to them.

The conference unanimously placed the unborn baby on the child protection register under the category of likelihood of physical injury. The conference was concerned that Colm could possibly harm the unborn baby by the repeated physical assaults on Chloe while still pregnant, but would undoubtedly pose a considerable threat to a new baby, as Colm was convinced that Chloe had become pregnant by someone else.

The child protection plan was as follows:

Case history 5.1—cont'd

- *Safeguard the child from future harm*. This was achieved by providing Chloe with alternative accommodation 20 miles away in the city. The domestic violence unit placed an alarm in the house should Colm track her down. An injunction against Colm was taken out through the courts to ensure Chloe's safety. Any breach of the conditions would ensure that Colm could be arrested, should he be seen anywhere near the house.
- *Promote the child's health and development*. Chloe was to be encouraged to attend for antenatal care, and provision for this was to be achieved safely without interference from Colm. In this respect social services arranged for Chloe to be accompanied and driven to these appointments and returned safely. The health visitor visited more regularly than usual, and offered help, support and encouragement.
- *Support the family to promote the welfare of their child provided that it is in the best interest of the child*. Chloe's mother was supported to travel to Chloe's new accommodation to help her daughter and impending grandchild. She was also to be a protective factor should Colm find out where Chloe was living.
- *Plan the work to be carried out in order to achieve de-registration*. Any conference following an initial child protection conference is called a **review child protection conference** and this must be within 3 months of the initial child protection conference. If it is considered that the child is no longer at continuing risk of significant harm that requires safeguarding then the review conference can decide that registration on the child protection register is no longer necessary.

Chloe gave birth safely to her daughter, Lily, at 38 weeks of pregnancy. She remained in her new accommodation postnatally but decided to move back, with Lily, to the town where she had been studying at university and where she had good friends. She settled in well and has had no further contact with Colm, who had drifted to a new city himself and had not been seen for a long time. The review child protection conference unanimously agreed to de-register Lily from the child protection register as the child protection plan had been successful and Lily was well cared for, loved and not at any risk of significant harm.

THE CORE GROUP

The core group will meet within 10 working days of the initial child protection conference. The group will consist of the key worker, the family members and the relevant professionals. Midwives would normally only be invited to be a member of the core group if the child protection conference was on an unborn baby; such as the midwife's crucial involvement with Chloe's pregnancy. If a child protection conference is convened around the time of birth, or postnatally, then you may be invited to the conference because your input and knowledge of the family are essential for the conference to reach a decision. However, it would be unusual for you to be involved with the core group, as your professional input to the family will soon be concluded.

In any child under school age the health visitor is an essential professional for any core group and it would be unusual for the health visitor not to be part of this process. She therefore has knowledge of such procedures and how they work and is an excellent resource for you, so that your knowledge of both the family in question and child protection procedures can be enhanced. It would be beneficial for you to use her expertise to enlighten and extend your own.

AN OUTLINE OF INFORMATION CONTAINED IN THE REGISTER

– The child's name, address, gender, date and place of birth
– Where the child is living
– The legal status of the child
– Full names of the parents or carers and regular visitors to the household and their relationship with the child
– Full names, dates of birth and gender of other children in the household
– Full name of the known or suspected abuser of the child

– Date of referral to a statutory agency and the source of the referral
– Category of abuse under which the child is registered

– Name and contact number of key worker
– Other agencies providing services to the child and family
– GP's name, address and contact number
– Health visitor's name, address and contact number
– Child's school, playgroup, nursery or childminder including a contact number

– Date of registration and the child protection plan
– Date when carers/parents were told of the registration and the child protection plan
– Date of review conference
– Record of all enquiries to the register

The register must be kept up to date and confidential unless the information is needed for a legitimate enquiry. The register should be accessible at all times for such enquiries. Details of enquirers are always checked before information is given.

If such an enquiry reveals that the child is registered then the name of the key worker is given. If an enquiry were made about a child living at the same address as a registered child then this information would be passed to the key worker.

If an enquiry reveals that the child is not on the register, then the information is recorded together with the advice given to the enquirer. If a second enquiry were made about the same non-registered child then the enquirer will be told that previous enquiry had been made and a referral should be made to social services as a potential child in need.

The Department of Health keeps a list of all custodians of child protection registers in England and Wales and should be notified of any changes in custodians. In Scotland a list of current keepers of the register is held by the Scottish Office social work services group in Edinburgh and they can be telephoned (0131 244 5486) for an up to date list or to advise on any local changes. This office also keeps contact points for all registers in other parts of the UK.

CATEGORIES FOR CHILD PROTECTION REGISTRATION

As previously mentioned a child or an unborn baby can only be placed on the child protection register following an initial child protection conference. All children on the register have a child protection plan for their unresolved child protection issues. If the child's name is placed on the register then the reasons must be clearly explained to the parents. It is not your role to inform parents, it is the duty of social services to undertake this task. The parents will be fully informed about the child protection plan and what is expected of them.

You will find that there will be leaflets available for the parents, which will be given to them by social services. These leaflets explain the processes that the parents are involved in. The NSPCC has a 24-hour free child protection helpline which can give advice (telephone 0808 800 5000) and they also produce leaflets which can be helpful to parents (see the section on the NSPCC in Chapter 7 for more information).

The conference members will be asked individually whether they feel that the child or unborn baby should be registered on the child protection register using the criteria documented above. If the members feel that registration is necessary they will also be asked under which criteria and with reasons for their decision. Children can be registered under more than one category; however, in reality, most conferences prefer to register under a single category. The chair will make the final decision on the category for registration. The category helps any enquirer to the register to determine the nature of the concerns on the child.

The categories on the register in England and Wales are as follows ('Working Together', 1999).

Physical abuse

Physical abuse may involve hitting, shaking, throwing, poisoning, burning or scalding, drowning, suffocating or otherwise causing physical harm to a child. Physical harm may also be caused when a parent or carer feigns the symptoms of, or deliberately causes ill health to a child that they are looking after. The situation is commonly described as factitious illness by proxy or Munchausen's syndrome by proxy.

Emotional abuse

Emotional abuse is the persistent emotional ill treatment of a child such as to cause severe and persistent adverse effects on the child's emotional development. It may involve conveying to children that they are worthless or unloved, inadequate or valued only insofar as they meet the needs of another person. It may feature age or developmentally inappropriate expectations being imposed on children. It may involve causing children frequently to feel frightened or in danger, or the exploitation or corruption of children. Some level of emotional abuse is involved in all types of ill treatment of a child, although it may occur alone.

Sexual abuse

Sexual abuse involves forcing or enticing a child or young person to take part in sexual activities, whether or not the child is aware of what is happening. The activities may involve physical contact, including penetrative (e.g. rape or buggery) or non-penetrative acts. They may include non-contact activities, such as involving children in looking at, or in the production of, pornographic materials or watching sexual activities, or encouraging children to behave in sexually inappropriate ways.

Neglect

Neglect is the persistent failure to meet a child's basic physical and/or psychological needs, likely to result in serious impairment of the child's health or development. It may involve a parent or carer failing to provide adequate food, shelter or clothing, failing to protect a child from physical harm or danger, or failure to ensure access to appropriate medical care or treatment. It may also include neglect of, or unresponsiveness to, a child's basic emotional needs.

In Scotland the categories are slightly different and are as follows ('Protecting Children', 1998).

Physical injury

Actual or attempted physical injury to a child, including the administration of toxic substances, where there is knowledge, or reasonable suspicion, that the injury was inflicted or knowingly not prevented.

Sexual abuse

Any child may be deemed to have been sexually abused when any person(s), by design or neglect, exploits the child, directly or indirectly, in any activity intended to lead to the sexual arousal or other forms of gratification of that person or any other person(s) including organised networks. This definition holds whether or not there has been genital contact and whether or not the child is said to have initiated, or consented to, the behaviour.

Non-organic failure to thrive

Children who significantly fail to reach normal growth and developmental milestones (i.e. physical growth, weight, motor, social and intellectual development) where physical and genetic reasons have been medically eliminated and a diagnosis of non-organic failure to thrive has been established.

Emotional abuse

Failure to provide for the child's basic emotional needs such as to have a severe effect on the behaviour and development of the child.

Physical neglect

This occurs when a child's essential needs are not met and this is likely to cause impairment to physical health and development. Such needs include food, clothing, cleanliness, shelter and warmth. A lack of appropriate care, including deprivation of access to health-care, may result in persistent or severe exposure, through negligence, to circumstances which endanger the child.

Physical abuse causing physical harm and subsequent injury to a child may be the easiest abuse to recognise. Bruises and burns can be seen on the child and without an adequate explanation as to how the child became injured then alarm bells would normally start ringing. Other physical abuse such as throwing, poisoning or drowning may not leave external signs of the abuse. Victoria Climbié was regularly made to sit tied up in a bath, which constitutes physical abuse. However, without the other injuries found on her then this form of abuse in itself may not have been recognised by any external signs.

Factitious illness by proxy is more difficult to recognise and it may be some time before all the factors show this to be the case, as illustrated in Case history 5.2.

Case history 5.2

Kirsty was expecting her third baby. Her first baby had been born normally at term. She had her second baby at 29 weeks and she induced this labour herself by inserting a knitting needle into her vagina and rupturing the membranes and then pushing continuously until the uterus was seen at the introitus. The baby was obviously cared for, once born, on the neonatal intensive care unit where he thrived and gained weight and was ultimately discharged home well and healthy. In the event physical harm was inflicted on this baby by the nature of his premature birth. Consequently the baby, once solely in his mother's care, had multiple admissions to the paediatric ward and into A&E with 'abdominal pains'. The little boy underwent invasive investigations and

---

Continued

Case history 5.2—cont'd

was regularly administered drugs in order to alleviate his 'pain'. It was not until someone pieced the whole picture together, and made a correct diagnosis of factitious illness by proxy, that the little boy was then rescued from this persistent trauma.

During this third pregnancy Kirsty had had 16 admissions to the maternity unit with 'possible SRM' or 'abdominal pain'. Each time she received large doses of pethidine to abate the 'pain', which Kirsty was very skilled at feigning. On the 16th admission a midwife voiced her concerns through the appropriate child protection channels and an urgent strategy meeting was called to assess the situation. The gathering of professionals at the meeting revealed that Kirsty had been feigning illness in herself to three different units in the area. In addition, all the units that Kirsty had been admitted to gave the same history – that Kirsty was inserting a knitting needle into her vagina to try and induce the labour.

A social worker visited Kirsty at home regularly to try and make some sense of the situation and to carefully explain to Kirsty the child protection procedure that was to be followed, in order to safeguard her unborn baby. The social worker explained that a child protection conference would be convened because of the risk to this unborn child. Kirsty found this news extremely shocking, particularly when the decision was made at the conference to register the unborn baby, under the category of likelihood of physical abuse.

The child protection plan, which was formulated at the conference, involved a psychological assessment of Kirsty's mental health. A robust system of support was put in place in order to support Kirsty through the traumas she had herself endured in life, and to try and reconcile some of the issues. Kirsty, with such support, did not try and induce labour again but went into spontaneous labour at 39 weeks and gave birth to a healthy baby which was discharged home with her. Careful follow-up and monitoring continued from different agencies postnatally and the baby was de-registered at the review child protection conference.

Meanwhile because Kirsty's history had surfaced and all the details were now on her and her children's medical records, further monitoring was able to take place should the situation decline again. Any deterioration would be picked up very quickly. In addition, Kirsty knew how to access help should she herself feel that she was slipping into her old habits again.

Emotional abuse, the persistent ill treatment of a child, can be much more difficult to see. Emotional abuse can be either acts of commission, where the abuse is deliberate, or omission, where the child is emotionally neglected as a result of inadequate parenting. Sadly, the failure to recognise emotional abuse can be much more damaging to the child in the long term.

It is unusual for babies, within the age we deal with, i.e. less than 4 weeks old, to be subjected to sexual abuse; however, there are some reported cases of this happening. Such cases are more likely to be where a male adult has masturbated over the baby's genitals rather than an act of penetration. The fact that the baby is not aware of what is happening does not detract from the fact that it remains an act of sexual abuse of that baby.

Acute neglect of a baby can be easy to see rather than the daily failure to care for a child's basic requirements such as feeding or caring adequately for him, as illustrated in Case history 5.3.

Case history 5.3

Carol was 17 when she gave birth to her first baby. She lived with Paul who had a violent temper and regularly hit Carol with a studded belt. Carol loved Paul; she said that he protected her and felt that he was showing his emotions when he hit her. Carol could always give explanations as to why Paul was violent towards her and felt that it was her fault. When the couple were first home with their baby Carol would care for the baby, but if Paul demanded attention then she would neglect the baby in order to meet his needs as she felt that Paul should always come first. On several occasions the baby had had to wait for food or for basic personal care, such as having a nappy changed. After a particularly stormy argument Paul walked out of the flat, much to Carol's distress. When he had not returned a couple of hours later she went searching the streets for him. The police were alerted to an incident when they received a message that a baby had been heard crying in Carol and Paul's flat for several hours. The neighbour who reported this stated that they felt that the child had been left in the flat alone. When the police arrived this was found to be the case.

The baby was removed by the police and taken into police protection. In such circumstances the police always inform social services and from this social services gathered further information about the couple. At this point the likelihood of ongoing significant harm to the baby could not be substantiated and Carol was extremely remorseful for what had happened and promised that it would never happen again. She received a police caution for the incident.

Two weeks later Paul went to visit his social security office for an appointment at 10 o'clock in the morning, stating to Carol that he would be back in a couple of hours. When he had not returned by the middle of the afternoon Carol started becoming anxious. By 6 o'clock in the evening she was extremely anxious and went to look for Paul with the baby in a pushchair. At 10 o'clock in the evening the police were called to a screaming, apparently abandoned baby that had been left outside a public house. The baby was again taken into police protection and social services were immediately informed.

This time an emergency protection order was secured by social services and the baby remained in a place of safety. A child protection conference was swiftly convened and the baby was placed on the child protection register under the category of 'neglect'.

Continued

Case history 5.3—cont'd

The circumstances following these incidents were clearly 'neglect'. It is not always so easy to define this category if it is as a result of persistently failing to meet the baby's basic physical needs. More time may be needed to build up a fuller picture over a longer period of time.

Carol and Paul's baby never returned home to them, as work undertaken with the parents repeatedly showed that Carol would not leave Paul, and that she would consistently put his needs before those of her baby. Neither Paul nor Carol was willing to work with social services or accept any support that could be made available to them. Ultimately a care order was obtained, through the courts, in order to keep the baby safe. Eventually the baby was released for adoption. The review child protection conference de-registered the baby, as the baby, having been accommodated safely elsewhere, was not in any further danger of being neglected.

DECISIONS ON DE-REGISTRATION OR CONTINUING REGISTRATION

Any conference that is held after the initial child protection conference is called a review child protection conference and de-registration must be considered each time. A child cannot be placed on the child protection register without a conference; however, there are certain occasions when a child can be de-registered without a conference. Nevertheless, it needs to be remembered that this situation is unusual.

The first review child protection conference should be held within 3 months of the initial child protection conference. Any necessary further review conferences, if the child remains registered, should be at intervals of not more than 6 months and continued for as long as the child remains on the child protection register. This is to make sure that the momentum for safeguarding the child remains in place and the child does not slip through its protective child protection plan.

The purpose of the review child protection conference is to:

- Review the safety, health and development of the child against the intended outcomes set out in the child protection plan.
- Ensure that the child continues to be adequately safeguarded.
- Decide whether the child protection plan should continue in place or whether it needs to be changed.

The review conference requires as much preparation and commitment as the initial child protection conference. If the child continues to be at risk of significant harm requiring ongoing safeguarding, then the child must remain registered on the child protection register. If it is considered that the child does not remain at risk of significant harm then the child can be de-registered. The core group has a collective duty to produce reports for the child protection review conference.

If the initial child protection conference is held on an unborn baby then you are highly likely to be a member of the core group, and therefore involved with the review child protection conference. If the initial child protection conference was held on a new baby then you would not be expected to be part of the core group or be invited to the review child protection conference.

In any event it would be unusual for a midwife to attend two review conferences because of the timescale of professional input we have with families. At the most you would attend an initial child protection conference and possibly one review conference. Initial child protection conferences tend not to take place early in a pregnancy anyway because (1) the baby is relatively safe in utero and (2) the woman may miscarry. If an initial conference is therefore convened at about 30 weeks then there is only usually time for one review child protection conference within your professional input time. The health visitor will have the ongoing duty to attend all the review child protection conferences.

A child's name may be removed from the register if:

• It is judged that the child is no longer at continuing risk of significant harm requiring safeguarding by means of a child protection plan (e.g. the risk of harm has been reduced by action taken through the child protection plan; the child and family's circumstances have changed; or re-assessment of the child and family indicates that a child protection plan is not necessary). Under these circumstances only a child protection review conference can decide that registration is no longer necessary.

• The child and family have moved permanently to another local authority area. In such cases, the receiving local authority should convene a child protection conference within 15 working days of being notified of the move, only after which de-registration takes place in respect of the original local authority's child protection register.

- The child has reached 18 years of age, has died or has permanently left the UK. ('Working Together', 1999: 5.93)

When a child's name is removed from the register notification is sent to all the representatives who were invited to the initial child protection conference. In this case you will get information about the ongoing well-being of the baby, either born or unborn, that you were involved with at that time. Sometimes you will automatically receive an invite to a review child protection conference just because you were on the original list of invitees. As already mentioned, in all probability you will not need to attend, particularly if you have had no further input with the family. In these circumstances get advice from a named child protection nurse or midwife and send your apologies, with appropriate reasons for non-attendance.

In some circumstances it may not be necessary to convene a review child protection conference for de-registration to occur, for example, a baby that has died or moved permanently to a foster home and will not be returned to the family. At such times the independent chair of conference may decide to write to all the original invitees to the initial child protection conference, outlining the new circumstances and suggesting de-registration. What usually happens is that the chair will ask for anyone who disagrees with the decision to de-register to write to them before a certain date with their area of concern. If no one objects then the child's name will be de-registered and a further letter will inform you of this decision.

Most families feel intense relief when their child is removed from the child protection register, as they can begin to have some control in their lives again. However, not all families welcome it and it should never lead to the automatic withdrawal of all help, as the family may suddenly feel vulnerable and alone. They may have felt understood, sustained and cared for by the relevant professionals involved in their lives; withdrawing all support could result in the situation declining and becoming a problem again.

The impact of these child protection processes on a family should never be underestimated. Any family caught up in such processes can feel undermined and angry; they may feel hurt and bruised for a long time, recovery can be slow.

ASK YOURSELF

---

1. What is the purpose of the child protection register?
2. What information is kept on the child protection register?
3. What are the criteria to work from when considering child protection registration?
4. What are the categories of registration?
5. What are the criteria to work from when considering de-registration?

REFERENCES

Department of Health (DH) (1999) *Working Together to Safeguard Children: A Guide to Inter-agency Working to Safeguard and Promote the Welfare of Children*. London: The Stationery Office.
Scottish Office (1998) *Protecting Children, A Shared Responsibility: Guidance on Inter-agency Co-operation*. Edinburgh: The Stationery Office.

FURTHER READING

Department of Health (DH) (2002) *Safeguarding Children in Whom Illness is Fabricated or Induced*. London: DH Publications (or available from the website *www.doh.gov.uk/acpc*).
Miller S. (2002) Child abuse and domestic violence. *British Journal of Midwifery*, 10(9):565–568.
Norfolk Area Child Protection Committee (2000) *A Guide to Inter-Agency Working to Safeguard and Promote the Welfare of Children*. Norfolk ACPC.
Stower S. (2000) The principles and practice of child protection. *Nursing Standard*, 14(17):48–55.

6

Serious case reviews

Serious case reviews (SCRs), also known as Chapter 8 or Part 8 reviews, are reviews of serious cases when a child has died and abuse or neglect are known or suspected to be a factor in the child's death. Serious case reviews are discussed in detail in, not surprisingly, Chapter 8 of 'Working Together'.

An SCR needs to consider whether there are any lessons to be learned from the tragedy and how well all the agencies involved with the case worked together. A serious case review would always be undertaken when a child dies from abuse but the area child protection committee (ACPC) may decide to commission a review if a child does not actually die, but has suffered from a potentially life-threatening injury, or serious and permanent impairment of health and development.

Recently there have been two highly publicised independent serious case reviews; the Lauren Wright enquiry and the Victoria Climbié enquiry, both will be discussed in more detail within this chapter.

It is important with such serious cases as Lauren Wright and Victoria Climbié that internal investigations are undertaken, even if an independent enquiry is to take place, to try and tighten up local practice, particularly if the enquiry reveals any failures in the local arrangements, to learn lessons from the tragedy. National lessons can also be learnt from local tragedies, as any highlighted local error could be occurring in other areas. The enquiry therefore hopefully prevents any further tragedies. Any necessary changes need to be made immediately rather than waiting for the final report, as there can be considerable delay between the tragedy and the publication of the report, particularly if the circumstances are complicated and involve many different agencies. Further changes may then need to be made once the report is available.

The purpose of a review is as follows:

- to establish whether there are lessons to be learned from the case about the way in which local professionals and agencies work together to safeguard children;
- to identify clearly what those lessons are, how they will be acted upon, and what is expected to change as a result; and as a consequence,
- to improve inter-agency working and better safeguard children. ('Working Together' 1999: 8.2)

Any agency or professional may refer a case to the chair of the ACPC if it is believed that lessons need to be learnt from inter-agency working. In Case history 6.1, a serious case review was commissioned by the ACPC about Emily and her baby son Tom. While in this case a child thankfully did not die, the potential was there and this was a 'near miss' of death for baby Tom. A serious case review was convened because of the seriousness of the case and for lessons to be learnt.

Case history 6.1

Emily was 16 and an IV heroin user. She injected prescribed heroin and in addition regularly used 'street' heroin. Emily also had an alcohol addiction and had regularly been admitted to a clinic to try and wean her off this addiction. She lived in an area where three maternity units were available. Women in this particular area would make their choice as to where they preferred to receive care and would regularly attend appointments and subsequent delivery in the unit of their choice.

Emily made it known to unit A that she wanted antenatal care and subsequent delivery there. Unit A and the corresponding community midwives were aware of Emily's history and supported her accordingly. Emily had a social worker because she had been a 'looked after child' (LAC) herself and had been in care. The health professionals looking after Emily felt satisfied that her social worker would be aware of any child protection issues and that this social worker would make the appropriate referrals, regarding protecting Emily's baby once born. Unfortunately these child protection procedures were not initiated.

When Emily went into labour she decided to go to unit B to give birth and duly arrived on the delivery suite. She appeared presentable and explained to the attending midwives that she had been shopping in unit B's area when she went into labour. The midwives took a history from Emily which appeared to be straightforward with nothing untoward and this story, not surprisingly, was believed. It is not an unfamiliar story for this particular unit, as it is within a main town, unlike the other two units.

Case history 6.1 — cont'd

Emily gave birth within a few hours and only needed some Entonox. She had a normal delivery, minimal blood loss and an intact perineum. Emily requested to go home directly from the delivery suite, with the female friend who had supported her throughout the birth. A routine paediatric check showed a healthy baby boy and Emily was hence discharged home. A message was sent via the correct channels to her community midwife in area A with details about the birth.

Emily's usual community midwife was on holiday and another midwife, oblivious to Emily's history, visited the next day. No one answered the door and the midwife left a note to say that she would visit the following day. This she duly did and again no one answered the door. This midwife became a little concerned and contacted the antenatal clinic at unit A to try and secure some information about Emily. The untoward history was thus imparted, creating immediate obvious anxiety for all these professionals regarding the health and well-being of the baby, once the situation became known.

A social worker and the police were immediately informed and they made a visit to the house, and the police enforced an entry. The baby was crying and in desperate need of food and attention. Emily had been injecting heroin and needles were scattered on the floor. There were several 'friends' in the house. The baby was taken back to unit B with police protection. The baby began withdrawing and needed medical attention for many weeks.

Recently the Department of Health commissioned some research into serious case reviews: *Learning from Past Experience – A Review of Serious Case Reviews* (Sinclair & Bullock, 2002). Some key messages were extrapolated from this work. Common themes, namely parental mental health problems and domestic violence, were regularly identified when a child became the subject of a serious case review. However, it was noted that the children's circumstances varied greatly. In some cases the abuse occurred out of the blue, in others it occurred in a context of low level need, and occasionally it arose in situations where it seemed to have been 'waiting to happen'.

Within these families some had prior involvement with agencies, often their whole lives from being children themselves to being parents had involved regular contact with agencies, and other cases were virtually unknown to any agency.

The government has a genuine wish to learn from the findings of child deaths or serious injuries and to improve the process for managing children at risk of harm. The media almost always make child deaths from abuse headline news and often make their own judgements from the details available to them, which may not always be fair or just in the circumstances. Acting as judge and jury before the full facts are known, particularly when sensational headlines are used, can have a devastating impact on workers involved.

Any review should highlight deficiencies in the system and the public have a right to this information, and details about where the system can improve. These lessons need to be learnt by professionals involved with the family in an equitable and honest culture, where professionals take some responsibility for mistakes made, but are not subjected to facing public humiliation at the hands of the media.

One of the earliest serious case reviews undertaken followed the death of Maria Colwell in 1974 from physical abuse (DHSS, 1974). There was a public outcry because the child protection system had failed Maria, and many professionals were blamed for not having done enough for her. The action plan from this enquiry was to guarantee that all the agencies involved with protecting children communicated more effectively, and that their actions in safeguarding children from physical abuse became more effective.

An official enquiry in 1987 carried out by Lady Butler Schloss (DHSS, 1988) into the allegations of sexual abuse of children in Cleveland, which was heavily reported in the media and press at the time, impacted on the formulation of the Children Act 1989 which was being produced at that time.

The aim of the outcome of serious case reviews becoming public is to lead to changes in law and professional structures. At present there are no readily available data on the number of serious case reviews that are undertaken; however, the Department of Health has recently introduced a computerised database of deaths or serious injuries of children, where there are child protection concerns. Local authorities are required to notify the Department of Health of any such cases, so that in future this information can be collated.

While there are no clear figures for serious case reviews, the Department of Health estimates that there are about 90 child deaths each year that are the subject of a full SCR.

Sinclair & Bullock (2002) explain that the new guidance from 'Working Together' (1999) on the undertaking of serious case reviews seems to be suggesting the following.

1. A change in emphasis from an inquisitorial perspective to a learning one. There would be less concern with whether guidance had been followed and more on lessons to be learned, particularly with regard to inter-agency working and the sharing of information.

2. In cases of serious injury, sexual abuse or maltreatment while looked after, clarity about why the review was being undertaken and what it would produce.

3. Clearer scope of the review from the outset, with the questions to be answered and the sources of information better delineated.

4. Clearer structures of both the reports from the welfare agencies and the ACPC overview and better information on key areas, such as the child's family history, family structure, previous referrals, decisions taken and work done.

5. A more robust action plan in which the responsibilities of each agency, the timescales and plans for implementation are specified.

6. Well prepared plans for the dissemination of reports and handling the media.

7. Reviews undertaken and completed within the suggested timescale, that is initiated within a month of the incident coming to the notice of the ACPC chair and completed 4 months thereafter.

8. The public availability of an executive summary report.

9. The setting up by the ACPC of an inter-disciplinary Serious Cases Review panel to consider whether a review should take place.

10. Evidence that reviews will increase awareness of child protection issues among local policy makers and practitioners.

Lessons should always be learnt from these reviews and some common themes seem to emerge with regularity.

• Failure to recognise any abuse which can be due to multiple reasons. A professional having contact with a family may not see or recognise abuse because it does not form the bulk of their work, such as a GP, health visitor or midwife, particularly if those individuals work in an area where such occurrences are unusual. A professional may not see any signs of abuse because the child is never seen by that individual, perhaps by parents not accessing medical care, or not allowing anyone to have contact with their child by denying access to the house.

• Communication is a major concern within any case review. It is common for many professionals to have had involvement with the family in question, all from different agencies and disciplines, and very little of this contact is divulged to other agencies. Professionals may communicate within their own discipline but not share the information outside it, consequently no one person takes overall control of all the relevant information. Record-keeping is another area that is prone to be below standard. Visits may be made to the family but the professional is not allowed to see the child and no record of this visit or any information is passed on.

• The common assumption that someone else would make a referral and then it does not get done. For example, a GP may send a child to A&E with suspicious fractures and assume that the doctor at the hospital would inform social services. In reality this presumes that the child will actually attend the hospital, if not then no referral will be made from that source. The child may attend A&E but the hospital doctor could be busy and again the referral does not get made by either doctor, the child easily slipping through the net. It is always better for two referrals to be made rather than none at all. In the case described above, there was an assumption that when Emily became pregnant child protection procedures would be initiated, because Emily already had a social worker. In fact, Emily's social worker was involved because of Emily's needs and not for the protection of her unborn baby. Different social workers, like most disciplines, have their own role with a client and they may not think about a separate aspect of care.

There are certain criteria to be met by independent writers of a serious case review. They must be:

• *Impartial*, no direct working contact or have had an operational role with the family.
• *Thorough*, all the factors need to have been considered and everyone involved given the opportunity to contribute.
• *Open*, nothing should be concealed or the integrity of the report will be undermined.
• *Confidential*, with due regard to the balance of individual rights and the public interest.

LAUREN WRIGHT

Lauren Wright was born on 16 July 1993 and died on 6 May 2000. Her stepmother and her birth father were found guilty of manslaughter and cruelty at Norwich crown court in September 2001. Lauren's stepmother, Tracey Wright and father Craig Wright were both jailed. Lauren ultimately died of a physical assault, having suffered long-standing physical and emotional harm. Being struck in her stomach so hard that her digestive system collapsed finally killed Lauren. She had more than 60 bruises on her body when she died, and only weighed just over 2 stone.

One month after the verdict in Norwich crown court, in October 2001, Norfolk Health Authority, on the instruction of the NHS, commissioned an independent health review on behalf of the stakeholders involved in the Lauren Wright case. Its purpose was to ask independent experts to examine the care that Lauren received from the NHS. This involved a detailed analysis of the actions taken by individuals and organisations providing care to Lauren and making an independent assessment of what happened.

The findings of the independent review were published in March 2002. Barry Capon, a solicitor and former chief executive of Norfolk county council, chaired the review. The review found evidence of poor practice and poor communication. The published report, available on the internet, quotes several factors which led to a situation where there was a failure to safeguard Lauren from harm.

The report made several recommendations including:

- Paediatricians in particular needed to improve their relations with other agencies, seek second opinions and avoid professional arrogance.
- Doctors should not be over reliant on other professionals, such as social workers and teachers to act in child protection cases, and the report called on the Royal Medical Colleges to improve training on the issues.
- Communication between agencies needed to improve.

The inquiry concluded that 'there was poor communication, failure to pursue diagnosis and over reliance on other professionals to act'.

Importantly, the review pointed out the absolute need for child protection training and that it was essential for all professionals engaged in services for children. The review clearly states that training 'is not an optional extra'.

Action plans have been drawn up since the publication of this enquiry to try and ensure that such a tragedy does not happen again. It is highly likely that there is a Lauren Wright action plan in your area, and it would be worthwhile finding out its recommendations for local action. Certainly in Norfolk, where Lauren died, there has been an extensive action plan and local implementation, which is being monitored by the strategic health authority of Norfolk, Suffolk and Cambridgeshire. Reports on the progress of the Lauren Wright action plan, within this strategic health authority, are available from the website: www.nscstha. nhs.uk.

One of the major repercussions of the death of Lauren Wright is that there is difficulty recruiting social workers in the areas where Lauren lived, and there are many vacancies, placing the remaining social workers under acute pressure. The president of the Association of Directors of Social Services said that the picture was 'grim'. She added that 'the net we use in order to catch and support children and families in distress is being stretched far too tightly. There is a very real danger of some of them falling through'.

Lauren Wright was not on the child protection register despite being seen regularly by social workers. Her stepmother Tracey Wright managed to explain Lauren's injuries as domestic accidents and fooled relatives, neighbours, teachers, social workers and paediatricians into believing that Lauren was merely a clumsy and sickly child.

VICTORIA CLIMBIÉ

Lord Laming's enquiry was published on 28 January 2003. This corresponds with the publication of this book and therefore the full impact of his recommendations are not yet known, but the reader would be well advised to keep abreast of the issues as the impact on child protection structures, both locally and nationally, will be significant.

The inquiry into the death of Victoria Climbié has been an extensive review of the child protection services, and Lord

Laming has promised that Victoria's suffering will mark a turning point in the care of vulnerable children. Ahead of the publication of this enquiry several proposals for reform were put forward in anticipation of Lord Laming's report. One proposal from the DH is the development of Children's Trusts as a way forward, bringing together social services, education and health into a single structure under the control of local government.

Victoria Climbié was part of a large loving family living in the Ivory Coast; she was the fifth child of seven children. Lord Laming described her, in a speech on 25 January 2003, as intelligent, articulate and enthusiastic. Her parents agreed that she should come to Europe to be educated. In 1998 her great aunt, Marie-Therese Kouao went to Abidjan and offered to take Victoria to live with her in France where she promised to give Victoria an education. Victoria arrived in Britain with Marie-Therese Kouao in April 1999. Within a year she was dead, killed by the people who had taken the responsibility of caring for her, namely Marie-Therese Kouao and her boyfriend, Carl Manning. Both of them are currently serving life sentences.

Carl Manning informed the trial that Marie-Therese Kouao would strike Victoria daily with a shoe, a coat hanger and a wooden spoon. She would hit her toes with a hammer and Carl Manning admitted hitting Victoria with a bicycle chain.

Victoria's final days in the depths of winter were spent living and sleeping in a bath in an unheated bathroom, in her own urine and faeces, bound hand and foot in a plastic bin bag.

Victoria was just 8 years old when she died of hypothermia on 25 February 2000 at St Mary's Hospital in Paddington. She had 128 separate injuries on her body.

Such cruelty is difficult to imagine but what is even harder is to try and speculate how it must have felt for Victoria.

Lord Laming was highly critical of the failure to protect Victoria by the agencies involved, namely police, health and social services, and described it as a disgrace. He concluded that the current legislative framework is fundamentally sound but there are gaps in its implementation. Lord Laming did not give most criticism to front-line staff but did concede that their performance often fell short of an acceptable standard of work. He placed the greatest failure with senior managers and members of the organisations concerned, whose responsibility was to ensure that the services provided to children such as Victoria were properly financed, staffed and able to deliver good quality services to children and families.

Lord Laming made 108 recommendations, expecting 46 of them to be implemented in 3 months and a further 36 in 6 months. He makes three basic propositions, namely:

1. A fundamental change in the capacity of the management in each of the key public services. The performance of each manager, and those in positions of leadership, must be judged by the quality of services delivered at their front door.

2. There must be a clear and unambiguous line of managerial accountability from top to bottom with no hiding place for managers if such a tragedy were to happen again. They must ensure that services are properly funded and adequately staffed to deliver services in a consistent and competent manner in order to reassure the public that children at risk will be safeguarded.

3. The current arrangements of area child protection committees, depending as they do on goodwill and best endeavours, should be replaced by a new national agency for children and families with powers to ensure that all the key agencies carry out their duties in an efficient and effective way.

Lord Laming continued that these objectives call for radical changes and recommends that a ministerial committee for services to children and families be set up at the heart of government. This committee would be chaired by a minister of cabinet rank and be responsible for ensuring that policies, legislation and departmental initiatives affecting children and families are properly considered, financed and co-ordinated. Reporting to this committee should be a new national agency for children and families responsible for advising on policy and practice at a local level and reporting to parliament on a regular basis on the quality and effectiveness of local services to children and families. The chief executive of this agency could take on the functions of a children's commissioner for England.

At a local level every local authority with social services responsibilities should appoint a committee for children and families, and members are to be drawn from each of the key services of education, police, probation, health, primary care, social services, etc.

Reporting to this committee must be a local board of management for services for children and families, chaired by the chief executive and with senior managers from each of the key services. This management board must identify the needs in their area and the resources available to meet those needs, and be accountable for the quality of the outcomes for children. A director of services for children and families must report to the board on the effectiveness of the services, the flexibility of the ways in which the resources are being used and the effectiveness of the inter-agency collaboration.

It is obvious from the above extract from Lord Laming's report that major reform is about to happen. It will involve major debate among key agencies for child protection, a bit like the debate and discussion of changes to our working practices when 'Changing Childbirth' (DH, 1993) was published.

One particularly sad comment from Lord Laming's report was that there were numerous occasions when the most minor and basic intervention on the part of the staff concerned could have made a material difference to the eventual outcome.

CONCERNS

The published reports on Lauren Wright and Victoria Climbié cause great concerns for the future of children's safety; however, the purpose of such reports (as already highlighted) is to air the issues and learn from the recommendations. Recently a joint report on the arrangements for safeguarding children with the title *Safeguarding Children* was published by the Department of Health (2002). This was not a serious case review rather a report of the inspection of services to protect children and involved inspectors from:

- the social services inspectorate (SSI);
- the office for standards in education (OFSTED);
- the commission for health improvement (CHI);
- Her Majesty's Inspectorate of Constabulary (HMIC);
- Her Majesty's Inspectorate of Probation (HMIP);
- Her Majesty's Magistrates Courts Service Inspectorate (HMMCSI);
- Her Majesty's Crown Prosecution Service Inspectorate (HMCPI);
- Her Majesty's Inspectorate of Prisons (HMIP).

The report makes a list of recommendations, which makes for useful reading as an adjunct to any serious case review.

It is important to remember that serious case reviews are not enquiries into how the child died or who is culpable, that is for the courts to decide. The enquiry seeks to identify where lessons can be learned, and how those lessons will be acted upon to safeguard children in the future.

ASK YOURSELF

1. What is the purpose of a serious case review?
2. Who was the subject of a serious case review in 1974?
3. What were some of the main findings from the Lauren Wright review?
4. What suggestions does Lord Laming make in his review of Victoria Climbié?
5. Think of any times in your career when a child may have been at serious risk of harm necessitating a serious case review.

REFERENCES

Department of Health (DH) (1993) *Changing Childbirth: The Report of the Expert Maternity Group*. London: The Stationery Office.

Department of Health (DH) (1999) *Working Together to Safeguard Children: A Guide to Inter-agency Working to Safeguard and Promote the Welfare of Children*. London: The Stationery Office.

Department of Health (DH) (2002) *Safeguarding Children: A Summary of the Joint Chief Inspectors Report on Arrangements to Safeguard Children*. London: DH publications (or Fax: 01623 724 524, or e-mail: *doh@prolog.uk.com* or at the website *www.doh.gov.uk/ssi/childrensafeguardsjoint.htm*).

Department of Health and Social Security (DHSS) (1974) *Report of the Committee of Enquiry into the Care and Supervision provided in Relation to Maria Colwell*. London: The Stationery Office.

Department of Health and Social Security (DHSS) (1988) *Report of the Enquiry into Child Abuse in Cleveland*. London: The Stationery Office.

Sinclair R, Bullock R (2002) *Learning from Past Experience: A Review of Serious Case Reviews*. London: DH (copies available from: Room 113, Wellington House, 113–155 Waterloo Road, London, SE1 8UG or Tel: 020 7972 4018; Fax: 020 7972 4627 or at the website: *www.doh.gov.uk/qualityprotects*).

FURTHER READING

Hall D. (2003) Child protection – lessons from Victoria Climbié. *British Medical Journal*, 326:293–294.

Wright D. (2002) We can't do it alone. *Community Care*, 25 April–1 May 2002:41.

7

Roles and responsibilities of different agencies

This chapter aims to give you some guidance about the different agencies involved with child protection procedures. An awareness and appreciation of the role of others is essential if you are to learn more about the processes and how your role dovetails in with others.

AREA CHILD PROTECTION COMMITTEE (ACPC) AND CHILD PROTECTION COMMITTEE (CPC)

Every area in England and Wales has its own area child protection committee (ACPC) and Scotland has its child protection committee (CPC). Both committees serve the same function and are an inter-agency forum for agreeing how the different services and professional groups should co-operate together to safeguard children in its area. It is a high powered committee made up of senior representatives of all the agencies involved with child protection: social services, the NSPCC (if active in the particular area), health, education, police, probation services, a domestic violence forum (if active in the area) and the armed services where appropriate.

The committees are committed to providing children in need of support with services that will protect them from harm, promote their health and welfare and minimise any adverse consequences of any abuse that they may already have suffered.

Other agencies become involved with the committee's work as needed, and will vary within each ACPC or CPC, for example, adult mental health services, child and adolescent mental health services, the coroner, the crown prosecution service, dental health services, drug and alcohol misuse services, or education establishments not maintained by the local authority. In addition, children's guardians, housing services, the judiciary, local authority legal services, prisons and youth detention centres, representatives of service users, representatives of foster carers, sexual health services, voluntary agencies providing help to parents and children, witness support services and youth offending teams (YOTS) may be involved.

In Scotland a core group of the CPC would most likely consist of local authorities (social work and education), police, health services, reporters to the children's panel, the procurator fiscal and the armed services if appropriate, such as in areas where large service bases are located.

Many ACPCs and CPCs find it useful and less unwieldy to have smaller subgroups that deal with specific tasks necessary for the smooth running of its functions, with these subgroups feeding into the main committee on a regular basis. The subgroups will vary according to the individual local requirements but a subgroup, for instance, may be set up specifically to look at the training needs for agencies within its own area.

The ACPC and CPC have an inter-agency responsibility for the development of local child protection policies and set out their own procedures and guidelines. There is an expectation that these policies adhere to the recommendations in 'Working Together' unless there is an exceptional local problem which justifies a variation.

The ACPC and CPC are expected to monitor and review the policies laid down by them, updating as necessary in line with, for example, the results of a public enquiry or a serious case review (SCR).

It is vital that you find out where the ACPC or CPC manual for your area is held, so that you can refer to it when necessary. The named individuals for child protection in your area should update this manual on a regular basis. It is usual for these policies to be accessible from the internet or your local intranet site. As well as the publication of policies on these sites there may also be a regular newsletter, so that you can discover what child protection issues are current in your own area. The manuals are not secret documents and are accessible to the public.

To avoid contradictory advice and unhelpful diversity among agencies, the committees should give a clear lead about how partnership with families should be developed to ensure a high standard of protection for children in their area (DH, 1995). This should be in ways that promote parental responsibility and strengthen their capacity to be able to protect their own children.

Every ACPC and CPC is required to publish an annual report and routine feedback to the committees should enable the committee members to judge the success of their policies, and to address any difficulties that may have arisen.

In a nutshell, the committees are bound by the relevant legislation, which is the Children Act 1989 for the ACPC, and the Children (Scotland) Act 1995 for the CPC. The committees are the driving forces in bringing together representatives from all the agencies that have a responsibility for the protection of children. In turn, all those representatives have a responsibility to ensure that they contribute fully and effectively to the work of the ACPC or CPC.

SOCIAL SERVICES

It is the responsibility of each local authority to prevent children in its area from suffering ill treatment or neglect through the provision of services under the Children Act 1989 or the Children (Scotland) Act 1995.

Social services are provided by the local authority and are expected to operate in accordance with local authority policies and the legal framework, and under the general guidance of the Secretary of State ('Working Together', 1999). Social services have statutory duties placed on them with regard to children. They must investigate reports of children suffering, or likely to suffer, significant harm and take the appropriate action to safeguard or promote the child's welfare. Social services take a lead role in child protection work but rely on the co-operation of all the other agencies involved. They manage key parts of the child protection process such as the initial enquiries to determine whether there are genuine concerns about a child, and if so they must enable appropriate meetings with other agencies within the required time frame. They are also responsible for the setting up of child protection conferences and the maintenance of the child protection register.

Referrals about a child's welfare reach social services from either the general public or a professional agency such as midwives. It has to be ascertained whether the referral is urgent, thus necessitating immediate action, or whether there are obvious concerns but the child is not in immediate danger. The social worker has a duty to investigate concerns following a referral and their duty is to:

- Make sufficient enquiries to ascertain whether and to what degree there is a risk to that child.
- Assess the child's needs.
- Decide whether and what action is necessary to safeguard and promote the welfare of the child.

These enquiries will also be initiated if a child has been taken into police protection and the police as a matter of course have informed social services.

This is a lot of responsibility for an agency to undertake and any social worker accepting a referral should have a team manager with specialist child protection experience to refer to, in order to be supported and advised appropriately.

Local authorities are obliged to protect children from any harm arising from abuse or potential abuse within a family, but must avoid unwarranted intervention, which is bound to be a difficult balance to achieve. They must have regard for the wishes and feelings of the child, parents and any other person who has parental responsibility. They must also consider the family's religious persuasion, racial origin and cultural and linguistic backgrounds.

The statutory child protection route that social services are obliged to follow is described in detail in Chapter 3.

In essence, social services have a statutory duty to co-ordinate and facilitate the services involved in protecting children. They have an obligation to provide services to keep a child at home unless there is immediate danger to the child and to provide the services necessary in order to achieve this. Parents and others can be under the mistaken belief that a social worker can remove a child from its home or its parents without any difficulty. This is not so, as no one has the power to remove a child from its home or parents without an order made in court.

THE POLICE

The police are involved in child protection as part of their responsibility for the prevention and investigation of crime. The police are a major part of the child protection procedures. They also have emergency powers not available to other agencies. They can without prior application to the court:

- Remove a child to suitable accommodation and keep him there.

- Detain a child in a place of protection, for example, keeping a baby in hospital and not allowing the parents to remove the child.
- Enter premises to search for a child in order to save life or limb.

Any child detained in police protection can be kept in a safe place within their protection for 72 hours in England and Wales and 24 hours in Scotland. This would give social services time to obtain a court order to continue the protection of the child, should this be necessary.

They can also:

1. Within a recovery order enter premises to search for a child in order to move the child into a place of safety, using reasonable force if necessary.

2. Arrest and detain an alleged abuser during their preliminary investigations. They can arrest without a warrant, if the arrest is necessary to protect a child from the continuation of abuse.

3. If an abuser is charged with an offence against a child, the police have the power to impose conditions on any bail that is granted, pending a court appearance, such as preventing the abuser having contact with the child. Such a condition may give the police permission to arrest that person if they have reasonable grounds to think that a breach of the bail conditions is being made. This should prevent the abuser from being able to have any contact with the child.

In any of these circumstances the police would inform social services as a matter of course. If a child is being kept in police protection the Children Act makes these conditions.

The designated officer shall allow contact with the child if, in the opinion of the designated officer, it is both reasonable and in the child's best interests. The people allowed contact are:

- The child's parents.
- Any person who is not a parent of the child but who has parental responsibility for him.
- Any person with whom the child was living immediately before he was taken into police protection.
- Any person in whose favour a contact order is in force with respect to the child.
- Any person who is allowed to have contact with the child by virtue of an order under section 34 (of the Children Act).

- Any person acting on behalf of any of those persons.

If a child is subject to police protection then the police do not have any parental responsibility for the child and could not therefore give consent for any medical examination on behalf of the child. However, they are expected to do what is reasonable to safeguard and promote the child's welfare.

It is expected that the police will inform as soon as possible those people who need to know that the child is in police protection including:

- The child's parents.
- Every person who is not a parent of his but who has parental responsibility for him.
- Any other person with whom the child was living immediately before being taken into police protection.

The police are not expected to accommodate a child on their premises, their role is to ensure that the child is cared for in an appropriate and safe place.

Most areas will have a specialised police unit dealing solely with child protection issues and all cases will be referred to the unit. This ensures a development of expertise and better communications with other agencies because of the identification of the key police officers dealing with child protection.

The police have a responsibility for dealing with the criminal aspect of an abused child and the prosecution of offenders through the criminal system. The police are always invited to child protection conferences and will usually attend unless they have knowledge in advance that there are no criminal issues that need to be addressed. This specialised police unit will work closely with social services as regards any child deemed to be at risk.

The role of the police within child protection differs from other police work as it deals with more than just pursuing a conviction of a suspected offender. Page (2001) says that what the police bring to child protection is their experience of conducting investigations to the high standard of proof demanded by criminal law. Indeed, evidence gathered in interviews by the police might subsequently only be used in civil proceedings instigated by another agency for the protection of the child.

Criminal proceedings demand that convictions should only be made if the evidence is 'beyond all reasonable doubt', whereas civil proceedings have a lower threshold, which is 'on the balance of probabilities'.

Whilst investigating allegations of child abuse the police will normally collect a considerable amount of information, irrespective of whether they decide to institute criminal proceedings. This information may be highly relevant in order to protect a child and should, where appropriate, be shared with other agencies.

THE NATIONAL SOCIETY FOR THE PREVENTION OF CRUELTY TO CHILDREN (NSPCC)

The NSPCC is a voluntary organisation and a registered charity dependent on public donations for its income. It is the UK's leading charity specialising in child protection and the prevention of cruelty to children. It is unique in that it is the only voluntary organisation that has been given statutory powers that can initiate any action necessary in order to safeguard a child at risk.

The mission statement from the NSPCC is:

To end cruelty to children. Our vision is a society in which all children are loved, valued and able to fulfil their potential. In other words, a society that will not tolerate child abuse – whether sexual, physical, emotional or neglect. (www.nspcc.org.uk)

The NSPCC is staffed by child protection officers, who are qualified social workers and who are supported by ancillary staff. The NSPCC has a 24-hour national child protection helpline, which is a free service providing counselling, information and advice to anyone, including children, concerned about a child's safety. In addition they have a bilingual Welsh helpline, an Asian helpline in the relevant language and a textphone service for people who are deaf or hard of hearing. The number to call is 0808 800 5000. The helpline is confidential and staffed by experienced social work counsellors. They can then, if appropriate, make a direct referral to the police, a local NSPCC team or the local social services department.

Anyone telephoning the helpline would not be identified to the family in question. However, it would be explained to the caller that if a child was genuinely perceived to be at risk then the NSPCC is obliged to divulge the information on a 'need to know' basis to those who have a legal responsibility to protect children from harm.

The NSPCC has a strong national voice campaigning for children's rights, needs and protection. The independence of the NSPCC allows for local needs to be considered when looking at assessment and therapy work. They organise drop-in centres for families, preventative programmes and training and consultancy work for professionals working within child protection. Many of their training courses are held at their national training centre in Leicester, which has residential facilities, but they will also run courses at a more suitable venue if it is more convenient.

The organisation's library service is a unique national resource for anyone working within child protection and child welfare. It offers the most comprehensive collection of reports, journal articles and other resources on these subjects in the UK. Visit 'NSPCC Inform' on their website, which gives direct access to the NSPCC library catalogue.

They have also produced an excellent series of leaflets; some speak directly to parents and some to children themselves. A few examples are:

- *Protecting your baby*: useful tips on coping with the pressures of caring for a baby, including how to get help if feeling pushed to the limit.
- *Get ready*: advice on preparing for the emotional demands of a new baby.
- *Handle with care*: advice on holding and handling a baby safely.
- *Encouraging better behaviour*: a practical guide to positive parenting.
- *Behave yourself*: positive ways of managing a child's difficult behaviour.
- *Home alone*: ensuring children are safe if left at home alone on their own.
- *Out alone*: advice on safety when children are out alone or with friends.
- *Putting children first*: a guide to young children's needs for parents of children aged 0–5 years.
- *Listening to children*: how to communicate more effectively with children.
- *Stop the violence*: a guide to keeping children safe from abuse.
- *Stress – a guide for parents:* useful tips for dealing with the stresses of caring for children.

- *Have fun and be safe*: choosing a leisure organisation with good child protection practices.
- *Are you worried about the safety of a child?*: useful tips on what to do if you are concerned about the safety of a child.

Many of these leaflets are obviously written for parents with older children but it is worthwhile having some knowledge of them.

A useful training and resource pack that is aimed at all health professionals but is particularly useful for midwives is called *'Fragile handle with care; protecting babies from harm'* which can be purchased from the NSPCC and gives a good basic grounding in child protection processes and procedures (see review in MIDIRS March 2002; 12(1):140).

Find out whether there is a local NSPCC team in your area. If so, make contact, spend some time with them, and further your knowledge in child protection through professionals who specialise in this field.

HEALTH WORKERS

Health professionals, including both community-based workers, such as GPs, midwives, health visitors, practice nurses and school nurses as well as hospital-based staff, are well placed to identify children at risk of being harmed. 'Working Together' says that nurses, midwives and school nurses must be provided with child protection training and must have regular updates as part of their post-registration educational programme. There is specific information regarding the role of the midwife. It says:

Midwives are involved with parents from the confirmation of the pregnancy through until some time after the baby's birth. As well as working with clients to ensure a healthy pregnancy and offering education on childcare and parenting, the close relationship they foster with their clients provides an opportunity to observe attitudes towards the developing baby and identify potential problems during pregnancy, birth and the child's early care. ('Working Together', 1999: 20)

Other health workers, who come into contact with vulnerable adults, should be alert to the possible risk to a child should one of their clients become pregnant, or if an assessment of a client exposes concerns that this particular adult may be a danger to a child.

It is essential that health workers collaborate together, where necessary, in order to safeguard children from harm.

'Working Together' lists other health professionals who provide help and support to promote children's health and many work with vulnerable children and families that experience problems looking after their children. All these health workers should be aware of the local ACPC or CPC procedures for protecting children:

- accident and emergency staff;
- ambulance service staff;
- clinical psychologists;
- dental practitioners;
- staff in GU clinics;
- obstetric and gynaecological staff;
- occupational therapists;
- physiotherapists;
- staff working in the private health-care sector;
- staff in sexual health services and pregnancy advisory workers;
- speech and language therapy staff;
- other professions allied to medicine.

In addition, nurses working in NHS Direct should have access to clear procedures, training and advice on child protection.

Many health professionals are in a position to offer positive health promotion, education and constructive intervention services to help reduce any predisposing factors. All these staff have a duty to acquire sufficient knowledge about child protection and know which channel of communication is needed and how to refer to a statutory agency if necessary. Health workers have no statutory powers but have a duty to care adequately for their clients in order to safeguard children at risk of harm. Health workers need to remember though that they have a duty to never delay in taking emergency action in order to protect a child.

Health workers should keep meticulous records in all circumstances and particularly if there are child protection concerns. DH (1997) says that the need for accurate, up-to-date, legible and complete records has never been more important. They confirm that this is essential where child protection issues are raised. Because of the nature of child protection it will be expected that this information is shared with others who need to know about the concerns; this would also include involving and sharing information with the parents. This would usually be after a full discussion with the named professionals in child protection or your manager, unless you have experience and specialist knowledge of child protection procedures.

The Department of Health (1997) publication *Child Protection: Guidance for Senior Nurses, Health Visitors and Midwives and their Managers* gives direction when dealing with hospital records. On page 20 under a heading 'hospital records' it says:

• Nursing records in hospitals are often shared with children and parents/carers. But records kept at the bedside are also accessible to others. Information of a confidential or sensitive nature, in particular child protection concerns, will need to be kept securely, even when it has been shared with the family.

• Where the sharing of concerns or information with parents/carers could put the child at further risk of harm the documentation pertaining to child protection matters should be kept separately from other nursing records and not be accessible to them.

• In these cases nursing documentation should include a record of significant family contacts, contacts with other health professionals and other agencies, outcomes of child protection procedures and any other legal orders in force.

• Local trust policy on secure storage and period for keeping records should be followed.

Any health professional who has been called to give evidence in court as a result of child protection proceedings would strongly sanction this information on record-keeping. Attending court can often be a long time after the event and any professional will rely on the contemporaneous records made at the time. If this record-keeping is poor then the evidence given will most likely be equally poor, as memories can fade, with subsequent disadvantage to the child. Very often it is the named professional who is called to court to give 'hearsay' evidence. She has not had contact herself but because of the sheer volume of midwives and nurses who have cared for the family while in hospital, it would be too unwieldy to request all those professionals to be called to court. Personal experience of trying to read illegible writing in the intensity of a court situation would beg everyone to take care with their record-keeping. It is also essential to write a date on each page and regular times, and to note how many days old the baby is in the records, as once photocopied they can very quickly get out of order and again this can lead the court to believe that they have a non-credible witness. The untoward repercussions for the child could be enormous. It would be dreadful to feel that a child's right to a secure life was sacrificed because of a poor standard of record-keeping.

DESIGNATED AND NAMED HEALTH PROFESSIONALS FOR CHILD PROTECTION

Each health authority has to identify a senior paediatrician and a senior nurse with a health visitor qualification to become the designated professionals that take a lead on all aspects of health services contributions across the health authority, both within primary care trusts (PCTs) and acute trusts, to safeguard children.

'Working Together' (page 18) says this about the designated professionals:

Designated professionals are a vital source of professional advice on child protection matters to other professionals and to social services departments. They will play an important role in promoting and influencing relevant training, skilled professional involvement in child protection processes in line with ACPC protocols, and participation in case reviews. They should comprise part of the local health service representation on the ACPC. The designated professionals will normally be based in a Trust, but will have responsibilities across the health authority area. In this authority wide capacity, they should establish regular contact with named professionals in Trusts (including Primary Care Trusts) . . .

It would be useful to know the names of the designated doctor and nurse within your own trust, as they are the most senior professionals for health workers that work within child protection procedures. These posts are usually full-time jobs and therefore the working days of these designated professionals are spent solely on dealing with child protection matters. In most circumstances information about child protection would be accessed through the named professionals within your trust and these named professionals would access further information from the designated professionals should this be necessary.

Each NHS trust (both acute and PCT) should have named professionals for child protection and these are the individuals that you need to know for help and advice with any child protection concerns. Some trusts, either acute or PCT, have a full-time named individual, but many trusts have named individuals that are also working in another capacity.

The named doctor would be a paediatrician in an acute trust and would usually be a hospital consultant paediatrician; in a PCT it would usually be a community consultant paediatrician or a GP. If your main work is in the community it is important that you know the named individuals both within the acute unit and your particular PCT. In addition to the named doctor within the PCT there will be a named nurse; this would normally be a nurse with a health visiting qualification. Both of these individuals would be an excellent source of information should you need it.

The named nurse within an acute trust may or may not have a midwifery qualification; they may have a paediatric background instead. Some trusts, such as my own, have a named nurse and a named midwife. The named individuals work together according to the age of the child. In any event these are the individuals with the specialist clinical expertise and knowledge to help you on child protection matters. They should have knowledge of the local arrangements necessary to protect children and have an important role in ensuring that fellow professionals and other agencies network well together in safeguarding children.

While this framework can be written here for you it is obviously important to understand the procedures within your own trust for child protection matters, as your local area may expect a certain line of action not actually covered here.

'Working Together' recommends that the named individuals within a trust take a professional lead on child protection matters and that these named individuals have expertise in local arrangements for safeguarding children and promoting their welfare. It is expected that they provide an important source of advice and expertise for fellow professionals and other agencies. They also have an important role in promoting good professional practice within the trust in order to safeguard children.

In essence the arrangements for safeguarding children within health organisations are centred on the named and designated individuals for each and every acute trust and PCT.

CHILDREN'S GUARDIAN

Children's guardians (formerly known as guardian *ad litem*) are experts who provide independent advice to the courts where there are legal proceedings involving a child. They are known as curator *ad litem* or 'safeguarders' in Scotland but the roles are similar.

They will have a social work qualification and work independently of social services. They are appointed by the court to solely represent the child and his best interests. As part of their duty the children's guardian will appoint a solicitor to act for the child in making recommendations to the court. They do not normally take part in the child protection process but may attend a child protection conference, as an observer, in order to gather as much information about the child's circumstances as possible.

The children's guardian has a right of access to see all the information and take copies of records held by social services or the NSPCC relating to the particular child. They may also interview any relevant professional, including health professionals who have had dealings with the child. This full information will be presented in court by the children's guardian in the form of a written report and questions will be put to the children's guardian regarding its contents and the conclusions reached. This guidance will be highly significant to the court and the decisions made because of the independence of the children's guardian who has taken no one's side but the child's. Lusk (1987) says that the children's guardian has a demanding role. She must have excellent communication skills and an ability to use her wise ear to pierce the truth and unscramble all the information laid before her in order not to take any side but the child's.

The Children (Scotland) Act says this:

> The use of safeguarders in children's proceedings gives added protection to children who come before children's hearings and the court in that they are appointed to represent the child's best interests in the proceedings – but not to act as an advocate for the child. The Act now requires children's hearings and the sheriff to consider in all situations the appointment of a safeguarder.

CHILDREN AND FAMILY COURT ADVISORY AND SUPPORT SERVICES (CAFCASS)

Children's guardians were formerly chosen from panels established by the local authority in accordance with the Children Act 1989. This was a service known as the guardian *ad litem* and reporting officer service (GALRO); however, GALRO has been brought under the umbrella of CAFCASS. CAFCASS has brought together the family court welfare service (FCWS, currently part of the probation service), GALRO and the children's branch of the official solicitor. CAFCASS has been established under the provisions of the Criminal Justice and Court Services Act 2000 (www.cafcass.gov.uk). The benefits of CAFCASS are:

• A more child-focused service, pooling the experience and expertise of the three services, and focusing on representing the needs, wishes and feelings of children in family proceedings.

• A service able to reflect today's diverse communities.

• A more professional service, highlighting and disseminating best practice, and ensuring continuous professional development of staff, so they are up to date with new developments, e.g. the consequences of the recent Appeal Court decisions on the cases involving domestic violence.

• A better service to the courts, based on the above points, and the greater adaptability and flexibility of a national service whose staff will increasingly be able to work across the current professional boundaries between court welfare and guardian work.

• A more visible and accountable service, being a national service with a voice in the development of policy and a service open to independent inspection and audit and accountable, through the Lord Chancellor, to parliament for its performance.

• CAFCASS will also be available to support parents who are bringing proceedings to the family courts because they are in conflict over the arrangements for their children or finances.

This creation of CAFCASS represents a major organisational change merging 54 FCW services, 57 GALRO panels and the official solicitor into one. This new organisation seeks to continue to develop and improve the service and move gradually towards more flexible and generic styles of working so that there is unity of the service across boundaries.

SOLICITORS

According to the complexity of the child protection case, the spectrum of solicitor involvement would range from no involvement to many solicitors being involved, representing different clients. Solicitors who may be involved and their duties are as follows.

1. A local authority solicitor who is employed by the local authority. Their client in the child protection procedures is the

social services department of the local authority. The social services department will ask the local authority solicitor for advice on whether or not a particular case reaches the criteria for requesting a court to make an order to protect a child through the courts. The local authority solicitor will attend meetings and will continue to advise social services on the legal aspects of the case and should prepare and submit witness statements to the court. They will attend court representing social services and are under a duty to present the case fairly by disclosing all relevant information to other solicitors involved, whether or not they intend to use it.

2. The parents' solicitor (this may be one solicitor for both parents or a separate solicitor for each) would usually specialise in court work and particularly family law. The parents would have chosen this solicitor and this would usually be a solicitor who is a member of the law society's children's panel. The Citizens Advice Bureau keeps information regarding solicitors who specialise in this aspect of law. The parents are automatically entitled to legal aid in childcare cases, so do not have to directly pay for this representation. The duty of the parents' solicitor is to advise the parents before any hearing, help them prepare statements of their evidence, and interview and take statements from any witnesses. The solicitor represents the parents in court, introduces their evidence and cross-examines any witnesses on any points on which their client disagrees.

3. The child's solicitor acts for the child but usually takes instructions from the children's guardian, unless the child is mature enough to instruct the solicitor in his own right. This solicitor works closely with the children's guardian, advising on the legal aspects of the case. Together they discuss and agree what further expert evidence needs to be obtained on behalf of the child.

Child protection proceedings in court in England, Wales or Scotland are held in private; the identity of the child is confidential to the court. The court is not open to the public or observers, unless an observer would benefit the court. No information would ever be disclosed in the media.

ASK YOURSELF

---

1. What is the main function of the Area Child Protection Committee (ACPC) and Child Protection Committee (CPC)?
2. Who has a statutory duty to co-ordinate and facilitate the protection of children?
3. What, in essence, does this duty comprise?
4. What role do the police have within child protection procedures?
5. What immediate powers to safeguard a child from harm are available to midwives?
6. What is the function of the NSPCC?
7. Name any other health workers and their role that may be involved with the child protection process.
8. Who would be appointed by the court to solely act in the best interests of a child?
9. What role do solicitors have in child protection?

REFERENCES

Department of Health (DH) (1995) *The Challenge of Partnership in Child Protection: Practice Guide*. London: The Stationery Office.

Department of Health (DH) (1997) *Child Protection: Guidance for Senior Nurses, Health Visitors and Midwives and their Managers*, 3rd edn. London: The Stationery Office.

Department of Health (DH) (1999) *Working Together to Safeguard Children: A Guide to Inter-agency Working to Safeguard and Promote the Welfare of Children*. London: The Stationery Office.

Lusk A. (1987) Dilemmas of the guardian *ad litem. Adoption and Fostering*, 11(4):29–31.

Page M. (2001) Police involvement in child protection. In: Polnay J. (ed.) *Child Protection in Primary Care*. Oxon: Radcliffe, Chapter 10.

Scottish Office (1998) *Protecting Children, A Shared Responsibility: Guidance on Inter-agency Co-operation*. Edinburgh: The Stationery Office.

FURTHER READING

Department of Health (DH) (1989) *An Introduction to the Children Act 1989*. London: The Stationery Office.

Scott L. (2002) Child protection: the role of communication. *Nursing Times*, 98(18):34–36.

Scottish Office (1995) *Scotland's Children: A Brief Guide to the Children (Scotland) Act 1995*. Edinburgh: The Stationery Office.

Simpson D. (1999) The midwife's role in child protection. Part 2: Practical matters. *The Practising Midwife*, 2(4):32–35.

8

The legislative framework

This chapter will look at the legislation governing childcare law in the UK. The significant statute for England and Wales is the Children Act 1989 and for Scotland it is the Children (Scotland) Act 1995. The guiding principles of both these Acts are the same; however, there are some variations between these two Acts within the processes and court orders, and they will therefore be dealt with separately in this chapter.

THE CHILDREN ACT 1989

The Children Act 1989 came into force in England and Wales on 14 October 1991. It is the most important reform in childcare law regarding children to have taken place in these countries for about 25 years. It has made the legal aspects of protecting children quicker, simpler and easier to use. The Act is long but the Stationary Office have printed a book called *An introduction to the Children Act 1989* (1989) which makes for less daunting reading. This particular Act is often wrongly referred to in publications as the Children's Act.

The Act and the rules, regulations and guidance that flow from it have a number of key themes, which can be summarised as follows:

1. They make children's welfare a priority;
2. They recognise that children are best brought up within their families wherever possible;
3. They aim to prevent unwarranted interference with family life;
4. They require local authorities to provide services for children and families in need;
5. They promote partnership between children, parents and local authorities;
6. They improve the way courts deal with children and families;

7. They give rights of appeal against court decisions;
8. They preserve the rights of parents when children are being looked after by local authorities;
9. They aim to ensure that children looked after by local authorities are provided with a good standard of care.

One major reform since the Children Act is the guiding principle that the best place for children to be brought up and cared for is within their own family. It seeks to minimise state interference in the care of children by introducing the 'no order' principle. The court will therefore only make an order if it is satisfied that to do so is positively going to benefit the child. Court proceedings can be lengthy and delays are commonplace. The Act presumes that delay is harmful to the child and should be avoided. The court is expected to draw up a timetable to ensure that the case is ready for a final hearing as quickly as possible and to take appropriate measures to reduce delay.

Before a court makes a decision as to whether to make a court order affecting a child, all sides of the case should be heard. The court has wide powers to make orders that in its opinion are best for the child, even though this may be a different order from the one requested by the local authority. If the court cannot be certain that an order will benefit the child then no order must be made.

The local authority, before ever getting inside a court room, must first of all do everything possible to help families stay together, providing that this is safe for the child. This may involve underpinning families with support, such as a home help, or finding a nursery place for a child. The provision of such services may mean that the courts do not need to become involved because of the support offered. Therefore the local authority may not apply for a court order if alternative systems for supporting vulnerable families are appropriate.

If the local authority makes the decision to apply for a court order then the court will expect to hear about any support that has been offered or has been established within a family. It would be unacceptable for the local authority to apply for a court order without having tried supportive measures for the family first.

SECTION 17 (S17)

It shall be the general duty of every local authority (in addition to the other duties imposed on them by this part) –

*a   to safeguard and promote the welfare of children within their area
who are in need; and*

*b   so far as is consistent with that duty, to promote the upbringing of
such children by their families, by providing a range and level of
services appropriate to those children's needs.*

If you have been involved with child protection procedures then
a reference to whether a case should proceed along section 17 will
probably have been discussed. Section 17 of the Children Act
gives local authorities a general duty to safeguard and promote
children remaining within their families, by providing an appropriate range of services. Partnership with the parents and joint
planning is the guiding principle. Section 17 processes are often
used when the parents are co-operating meaningfully with the
child protection process, with the agencies involved. Instead of
the forum for protecting the child within a child protection conference there would instead be a **family support conference**.

   Section 17 is not solely used for a child who is 'in need' because
of possible child protection concerns, this section states that a
child shall be taken to be in need if:

• He is unlikely to achieve or maintain, or have the opportunity
  of achieving or maintaining, a reasonable standard of health or
  development without the provision for him of services by a
  local authority.
• His health or development is likely to be impaired, or further
  impaired, without the provision of such services.
• He is disabled.

   Section 17 enquiries can move into section 47 enquiries at any
time if it is considered that the child is suffering or likely to suffer
significant harm, particularly if the parents stop co-operating
with the professional agencies. Section 47 is the full-blown child
protection route as outlined in Chapters 4 and 5 and more information about sections 17 and 47 can be found there.

SECTION 47 (S47)

Where a local authority –

a   are informed that a child who lives or is found in their area –
*   i   is the subject of an emergency protection order; or*
*   ii is in police protection or*

b *have reasonable cause to suspect that a child who lives, or is found,*
   in their area is suffering, or is likely to suffer, significant harm,

   The authority shall make, or cause to be made, such enquiries as
they consider necessary to enable them to decide whether they should
take any action to safeguard or promote the child's welfare.

Section 47 of the Children Act requires the local authority to make
such enquiries as they consider necessary to enable them to
decide whether they should take any action in order to promote
and safeguard the child's welfare. Such cases as outlined above
would be when:

1. A child is the subject of an emergency protection order.
2. A child is in police protection.
3. A child is aged under 10 years and in breach of a child
   curfew order.
4. There is reasonable cause to suspect that a child who lives,
   or is found, in their area is suffering or likely to suffer
   significant harm.

LEGAL RECOGNITION OF SIGNIFICANT HARM

Section 31 says:

The court may only make a care order or supervision order if it is satisfied –

a *that the child concerned is suffering, or likely to suffer, significant harm;*
   and
b *that the harm or likelihood of harm is attributed to –*
   i *the care given to the child, or likely to be given to him if the order were*
      not made, not being what it would be reasonable to expect a parent to
      give to him; or
   ii *the child's being beyond parental control.*

'Harm' means ill treatment or the impairment of health and development;
'development' means physical, intellectual, emotional, social behavioural
development; 'health' means physical or mental health; and 'ill treatment'
includes sexual abuse and forms of ill treatment which are not physical.
   Where the question of whether harm suffered by a child is significant turns
on the child's health or development, his health or development shall be
compared with that which could reasonably be expected of a similar child.

It is not possible to list all the circumstances that may result in
the likelihood of significant harm. This list is a reproduction of
the list in Chapter 4 and the following circumstances would normally indicate the need for a referral:

1. Any allegation of sexual abuse.
2. Parents whose behaviour may present a high risk to children because of:
   – domestic violence
   – drug and alcohol problems
   – mental health problems.
3. Physical injury caused by assault or neglect which requires medical attention, especially any injury to a baby under the age of 1 year.
4. Repeated incidents of physical harm that are unlikely to constitute significant harm in themselves but collectively may do so.
5. Contact with a person assessed as presenting a risk to children.
6. Children who live in a low warmth, high criticism environment which is likely to have an adverse impact on their emotional development.
7. Children who suffer from persistent neglect.
8. Children living in a household where there is domestic violence likely to lead to physical or emotional harm.
9. A child living in a household or having significant contact with a person convicted of an offence listed in Schedule 1 of the Children and Young Persons Act 1933 (a schedule 1 offender).
10. Children who may be involved in prostitution.
11. Other circumstances where professional judgement and/or evidence suggests that a child's health, development or welfare may be significantly harmed.

COURT ORDERS: THE CHILDREN ACT 1989
Emergency protection order (EPO)

This will only be made in extremely urgent situations when the child's safety is immediately threatened. The order places the child under the protection of the local authority for a maximum period of 8 days. The court may exceptionally extend the order for a further 7 days if there is reasonable cause to believe that the child is likely to suffer significant harm if the order is not extended.

An EPO can be discharged any time after 72 hours if an application is made to the court to do so, by his parents or carers, and the court is in agreement. An EPO will enable a child to be removed to other safe accommodation or, in the case of a new baby, keep the baby in hospital and not allow the parents to take the child home. This action gives the local authority time to reflect and initiate any action necessary for the future safety of the child. There is no right of appeal against an emergency protection order, but on expiry of the order there is no power to continue holding the child away from its parents or carers, and the child must be returned to them. If it is felt that the child needs to remain accommodated in a safe place then the local authority must return to court and apply for a care order.

It is not always necessary to keep a child away from home even if an EPO has been granted. It may be possible to have such supervision, within the home, which ensures that the child is safe there. Throughout the period of any EPO the parents or carers should, as far as possible, be involved in the discussions and planning for their child, or they should be kept informed of events if this is not possible.

Care order

A care order places the child under the care of the local authority. This again does not necessarily mean that the child has to live away from home but it does give the local authority power to exercise parental responsibility, which it shares with the parents. In the event of a dispute between the local authority and the parents over the arrangements for the child, the local authority would have the final say. If a child is under the auspices of a care order then the local authority has the power to remove the child from home or where he is residing, if necessary, without re-applying to the court. The care order lasts until the child is 18 unless the court discharges the order earlier, for instance, if the child's circumstances change so that the likelihood of significant harm has been resolved.

If an application for a care order cannot be dealt with in full because all the facts about a child are not known, an interim care order (ICO) can be made, provided that the court has reasonable grounds to believe, with the facts already available to them, that the conditions for an order are satisfied. An interim care order can last for up to 8 weeks, and can be extended by the courts for further periods of 4 weeks.

Generally where an application for a care order is made, the court will appoint a children's guardian whose duty would be to represent the child and safeguard the child's interests. The children's guardian has a duty to instruct a solicitor unless the court directs otherwise, or the court has already appointed a solicitor.

Supervision order

The local authority would apply for a supervision order if they were unable to form satisfactory voluntary arrangements with the parents to ensure the child's protection. This order places the child under the supervision of the local authority or a probation officer. A probation officer would not, of course, be involved with a supervision order on a baby. It does not give the local authority, or probation officer, any parental responsibility but it does give them rights of access to the child to ensure the child's well-being. The appointed supervisor has three specific duties:

1. To advise, assist and befriend the child.
2. To take all reasonable steps to ensure that the order is effected.
3. To apply for variation or discharge of the order if it is not working or has become unnecessary.

The appointed supervisor has the power to impose requirements upon those with parental responsibility for the child or any other person with whom the child is living.

A supervision order can last up to 1 year although it can be extended for a period of up to 3 years from when it was made. A supervision order cannot last beyond a child's 18th birthday.

Care and supervision orders differ in that the former places the baby into the care of the local authority, whereas a supervision order places him under the supervision of the local authority. The two orders are mutually exclusive. The local authority or authorised person applying for a care or supervision order must serve a copy of the application on every person who has parental responsibility for the child.

Child assessment order

This is an order that is used to cover non-emergency situations where an assessment of a child's well-being is needed. It would normally be used if the parents were not co-operating with the local authority by not allowing a request for a medical examination to take place; unlike an emergency protection order this can be appealed against. The court will specify on which date the assessment should begin and the order will remain effective for 7 days from that date and the court will decide the nature of the assessment. The courts would grant such an order if there were concerns about a child, usually physical concerns, and there was debate about how the condition came about. For example, a baby who regularly suffered broken bones or was often badly bruised and the picture was not consistent with non-accidental injury. A medical assessment could determine whether the child did have some underlying disease, which would rule out non-accidental injury. It is worth noting that a child assessment order is not very common and is not used very often.

POWERS AVAILABLE TO THE COURT

The court has a wide range of powers, which it may use after listening to all the evidence and may suggest an alternative to a care order. It may not support the local authority's application for a particular order. The more common alternatives to a care order are:

- A residence order to one of the parents or a relative with or without a supervision order to the local authority. A residence order requires a child to live with a specified person and if that person is not a parent then that person exercises parental responsibility for as long as the residence order lasts (usually up to the age of 16).
- A contact order which requires the child's carer to allow the child to have contact with a named person under any terms dictated by the court.
- A prohibitive steps order, which prevents a named person from doing certain things, which may affect the child, for example, having unsupervised contact with a child.

The court has the final say and may instead order that the child live with a suitable relative or friend rather than grant an order. They may also dictate that the child live with the non-abusing parent and prohibit anyone access to the child who poses a danger.

There is a right of appeal to a higher court to any party in the proceedings including the child. Under the Children Act appeals can be made against any order other than an emergency protection order.

PARENTAL RESPONSIBILITY

'Parental responsibility' means all the rights, duties, powers, responsibilities and authority which by law a parent of a child has in relation to a child and his property.

Married parents both automatically have parental responsibility. An unmarried mother has parental responsibility but an unmarried father does not. He can acquire parental responsibility by entering into a parental responsibility agreement with the mother or by an order of the court. Parental responsibility can only be taken away from the parents by the making of an adoption order. The local authority can only override the parent's responsibility by the making of a care order by the courts. The responsibility therefore of the local authority if granted parental responsibility is by reference to 'all the rights, duties, powers, responsibilities and authority, which by law a parent has in relation to a child . . .'. This is from section 3 of the Children Act.

The local authority gains parental responsibility through an emergency protection order, an interim care order or a full care order. This then limits the parental responsibility of the parents by these orders. Parental responsibility acquired through the courts will last as long as the order remains.

The only time that a parent loses all parental responsibility is when an adoption order is made and the parental responsibility then transfers completely to the adoptive parents.

THE HUMAN RIGHTS ACT 1998

The Human Rights Act means that for the first time in law there are positive guarantees of rights. Two Articles are of particular relevance to health professionals and they are Article 3 and Article 8 of the Human Rights Act.

Article 3 makes it plain that the guarantee is that no one shall be subjected to torture or to inhuman or degrading treatment or punishment. This has major implications for adequately safeguarding children's rights including their right to life (Article 2).

This means that all of us who are involved in any way with children need to consider whether our working practices are actually adequate in their arrangements for the safeguarding of children. If any public authority, midwives included, know of a child at risk of torture or inhuman or degrading treatment or punishment they have to take the appropriate action in order to avoid a breach of Article 3.

Article 8 deals with the right to respect for private and family life:

1. Everyone has the right to respect for his private and family life.

2. There shall be no interference by a public authority with the exercise of this right except such as in accordance with the law and is necessary in a democratic society in the interests of national security, public safety or the economic well-being of the country, for the prevention of disorder or crime, for the protection of the rights and freedom of others.

THE CHILDREN (SCOTLAND) ACT 1995

The Children (Scotland) Act 1995 marks a significant stage in the development of legislation on the care of children in Scotland. The Act is centred upon the needs of children and those needs are the central focus of the Act. It looks at families and defines parental responsibilities and rights in relation to children. The Act sets out the duties and powers available to public authorities to support children and their families and to intervene should the child's welfare necessitate it.

The essential principles and themes can be summarised as follows:

1. Each child has a right to be treated as an individual.

2. Each child who can form a view on matters affecting him or her has the right to express those views if he or she so wishes.

3. Parents should normally be responsible for the upbringing of their children and should share that responsibility.

4. Each child has the right to protection from all forms of abuse, neglect or exploitation.

5. So far as is consistent with safeguarding and promoting the child's welfare, the public authority should promote the upbringing of children by their families.

6. Any intervention by a public authority in the life of a child must be properly justified and should be supported by services from all the relevant agencies working in collaboration.

The guiding principle of the Scottish Act mirrors the Act for England and Wales in that the welfare of the child is the paramount consideration when his or her needs are heard in the court. No court order should be made unless the court feels that it would benefit the child. If a child is old enough then the court must take their views into consideration when making a judgement.

COURT ORDERS: THE CHILDREN (SCOTLAND) ACT 1995

Emergency child protection measures

The local authority, or any other person, can make an application to a justice of the peace for authorisation to remove a child to a place of safety or to prevent a child being removed from where the child is being accommodated, for example, not allowing a baby to be removed from hospital by the parents if there are child protection concerns. This application may not need to be heard in court as the justice of the peace can make an authorisation where certain criteria have been met. This authorisation only lasts for a maximum of 24 hours and a court order would therefore need to be granted to be able to keep the child in a place of safety.

If certain criteria are met then a police constable can give the authorisation to keep or remove a child within a place of safety without authorisation from the justice of the peace. This also only lasts for 24 hours.

Child protection order

A child protection order would be granted by a sheriff following an application from any person, should the child be at risk of significant harm. Anyone can apply for an order such as a teacher, doctor, police constable, relative or friend; however, in reality it is usually the local authority that makes the application.

The sheriff will grant this order only if they are satisfied that the local authority has reasonable grounds to suspect that the child is suffering or will suffer significant harm because of ill treatment or neglect. The sheriff will also want to be satisfied that the local authority are making such enquiries as will help them decide what action they should take to safeguard the child and that the parents are unreasonably denying access to the child.

The sheriff will want to know why such urgent action is necessary and whether it is in the child's best interests that the order should be made.

A child protection order may do things as follows:

• Require any person in a position to do so to produce the child to the applicant.
• Authorise removal of the child by the applicant to a place of safety, and the keeping of the child in that place.
• Authorise the prevention of the removal of the child from any place where he or she is being accommodated.
• Provide that the location of any place of safety in which the child is being kept secret should not be disclosed to any person or class of person specified in the order itself.

The sheriff will give directions as to how the order will enhance the child's welfare and will alter the directions when circumstances change. Notice of the making of the order must be given by the applicant to the principal reporter who, having regard for the welfare of the child, returns the child to his family, when, as a result of a change in circumstances, he considers that the child protection order is no longer justified.

A children's hearing will be heard at intervals to review the order and whether it needs to be continued. The children's hearing system is unique to Scotland. The hearing is made up of three individuals who have an interest in, and knowledge of children. They are all volunteers and do not have a legal qualification. The children's hearing may also deal with children who have committed criminal offences in addition to the children with welfare issues.

The children's hearing system is open to review and appeal and in these circumstances the sheriff would become involved. The sheriff is legally qualified and is the judge in the sheriff's court and can have an appellate role in deciding on an appeal from the children's hearing. Additionally the sheriff may be called upon to find that the grounds of referral have been established.

When the sheriff considers an application for a variation or to recall the order, the sheriff has the power to continue, vary (by giving new directions), or discharge the order.

Child assessment order

Only a local authority can apply to the sheriff for a child assessment order. It would be used to enable an assessment of the state of a child's health. It is similar to the child assessment order under the Children Act 1989, as it is not an order that would be made for emergency situations. If it is considered that (following the assessment of the child) the child needs protecting, then the sheriff must make a child protection order to secure the safety of the child.

The child assessment order would be granted if there was concern about the child's welfare and development and not enough information has been gleaned by the professionals to know whether action is needed to protect the child and consent has not been given by the parents for an examination.

The child assessment order ensures a proper examination of the child with minimum disruption to the child or the family. Depending on the outcome of the assessment it could lead to further child protection issues or reassure the local authority that such procedures are not justified.

Exclusion order

The order furthers the statutory measures available to protect children from harm or the threat of harm by excluding an alleged abuser from the family home. It prevents the person from entering the home, except with the express permission of the local authority. A person named in an exclusion order may be the child's parent or a member of the child's family or anyone from whom it is considered necessary to protect the child from significant harm or the threat of harm.

Only the local authority can apply to a sheriff for an exclusion order. The sheriff will consider the conditions that need to be met in order to grant the order. These are:

- The child has suffered, is suffering or is likely to suffer significant harm as a result of any conduct of the named person, such conduct being actual, threatened or reasonably apprehended.

- The order is necessary for the protection of the child.
- The order would better safeguard the welfare of the child than removing the child from the family home.

The sheriff may attach a power of arrest to the named person in the exclusion order. An exclusion order can be interim pending further information that would warrant a final exclusion order. The order will last for a maximum period of 6 months and is not renewable.

Parental responsibilities

The Children (Scotland) Act 1995 has laid down what a parent's responsibilities are. A parent must:

in the interests of your child and as far as practicable – safeguard and promote your child's health, development and welfare. Give your child the direction and guidance he or she needs. Keep up your personal relationship and contact with your child – even if you do not normally live with him or her. Act when necessary as your child's legal representative.

All mothers have these responsibilities and rights and only an order by a court can take them away. A father also has these rights but only if:

- He was married to his child's mother when she was pregnant.
- He has been given the responsibilities by a court.
- He has made and registered with the mother a parental responsibilities and parental rights agreement.

The parental responsibilities and parental rights agreement is a legal document showing that a mother who has parental rights and responsibilities and the child's father, who is not married to her, have both agreed that the mother should share her parental responsibilities and rights with the child's father. Only a natural father can sign the agreement, it cannot be a stepfather or the mother's partner who is not the actual father of the child.

The agreement once signed by both parents is then registered with the keeper of the registers of Scotland.

COURTS

Courts fall into different categories, starting with the simplest cases, which can be transferred upwards if necessary into higher courts. In England and Wales most child protection issues are dealt with in the magistrate's court and would only move into a higher court if the case became more complicated. In Scotland the children's hearing system would usually be employed for most child protection hearings.

Neither magistrates nor the volunteers for the children's hearing system have a legal qualification; however, there is usually someone available to give advice on legal points if necessary.

Higher courts would normally have a judge, or a sheriff who would be the judge in the sheriff's court in Scotland. The judge has a legal qualification and will hear evidence on more difficult cases. Particularly complicated cases concerning children, involving difficult legal issues, could be heard in the high court in front of a high court judge, in England and Wales.

Court proceedings involving children needing protection are confidential and held in closed court. No one other than the necessary parties will be allowed in to witness the proceedings. The closed court will decide whether or not to grant an order and direct the most appropriate way forward for the child. The court will listen to the evidence placed before it, from all the participants, and will make the child's future welfare its priority. The court is not concerned with finding guilty parties; this is a job for the courts that deal with criminal proceedings.

Criminal proceedings are entirely separate from care proceedings. In criminal proceedings the Crown Prosecution Service (CPS) decides to take the case to court after a police investigation. The court will decide whether the accused is guilty or not and then impose the penalty if necessary. The criminal courts do not decide about arrangements for children who have been subjected to abuse; they are dealing with the abuser. Criminal courts are not confidential and cases are likely to be published in the press. A parent who is accused of abusing their children may be attending both courts, one court to deal with the continuing safety and welfare of their child and the other to decide whether they should be charged with a criminal conviction.

It is unusual but possible for a midwife to be asked to give evidence in court. If you are asked to attend court, whether criminal or care proceedings, it is essential that you have a working knowledge of court procedures before attending.

Even with the improved timescale for hearings about children being heard there is often a delay between your involvement with the family and a court appearance. Recollections obviously fade, even though you may think at the time that the details will remain with you forever. It is therefore essential that your records are particularly thorough and as much detail is written down as possible. Make notes for yourself to jog your memory, such as the weather or any other incidental note to help you at a later date. Life in court is so much easier and more credible if the records are of a high quality and this cannot be stated enough.

A day in court can be slow and tedious with lots of waiting around. You should be given a specific time to attend rather than be expected to wait around from the start of proceedings, but in reality all kind of delays can occur. A previous case being heard may take longer than was anticipated or a vital witness or piece of evidence may be missing. Solicitors may make certain objections, thus slowing down the whole process. The proceedings may even be cut short if the outcome is clear at an early stage of the hearing. The hearing may be re-scheduled if a vital witness is missing. None of this helps, as you will most likely be feeling nervous. You will notice that the professionals used to attending court to give evidence will be prepared to wait, so take something to read with you or some knitting!

If you are called to court for care proceedings it will probably be following an approach from the local authority, usually from their solicitor. You will be asked to describe specific events and your observations of the parents' behaviour and maybe such things as the condition of the home. Quite frequently midwives will be asked to give an opinion upon the parenting skills of the parents or apparent injuries inflicted on the child.

The court will require a statement from you. If the order is being pursued as an emergency, then you may not have much time to prepare it, and in any event you will need the support of your named professionals for child protection or your manager. If there is a delay between your involvement with the family and your court appearance then you will have time to write your report and there is an acceptable format for doing this. Sometimes the local authority solicitor will take a statement from you and then it is signed once you are happy that it is factual and accurately reflects your facts and opinion.

The local authority is there to help and advise you; however, you will also need the support of a senior colleague experienced in the procedures, as the local authority solicitor will be busy with his own agenda, and will not be free to give you all the support and help that you may need. It is likewise important for you to have someone to de-brief with afterwards. You are allowed to make notes for your own benefit and to take records into court with you for reference, rather than just having to rely on your memory of events.

Childcare proceedings are less formal occasions than criminal proceedings. If the hearing is taking place in a higher court where robes and wigs are commonplace, these will not be worn during care proceedings. This is obviously less concerning should an older child be in court for the proceedings. The parties involved usually sit around large tables with most parties at the same level. The witnesses can stay seated to give evidence and the solicitors also remain seated when asking you questions. Remember that you are not on trial here, the focus remains at all times on the future well-being of the baby or child.

You may be challenged if your account of events is disputed or perceived differently by someone else; however, childcare proceedings are not meant to be unduly adversarial.

Some general advice about coping in court:

- Always tell the truth.
- Keep to facts only unless specifically asked for an opinion.
- Listen carefully to questions.
- Answer as clearly as possible.
- Think before answering questions.
- Do not waffle!
- If you make a mistake, then say so, do not try and cover it up.
- Always ask for a question to be repeated or said in a different way if necessary.
- Be prepared to say that you do not understand or you do not know.
- Do not bluff, you will be caught out immediately.
- Deal with one question at a time.
- Try not to anticipate the next question.
- Try not to overreact, stay calm, measured and in control.
- Do not let yourself be taken away from your own area of expertise.

If you are asked to attend the criminal court as a witness, for example, you saw a parent strike their child, then this will not be confidential and will be in open court. The welfare of the baby is not the focus of the criminal court; it is to decide whether the accused is guilty of the alleged offence. Solicitors or barristers for the defence and the prosecution will cross-examine you. The prosecution will try and prove the guilt of the parent and the defence will act on behalf of the parent and try and prove their innocence, this is usually by trying to discredit your evidence. Whatever happens, it is not you personally under attack, even though it may feel like it; it is simply the way that the law works.

ASK YOURSELF

1. What are the key themes that emerge from the Children Act 1989 and the Children (Scotland) Act 1995?
2. How would you describe significant harm?
3. List some of the circumstances that may make you suspect that a child may be at risk of significant harm.
4. What court orders may the court impose that can protect a child from harm?
5. Who has parental responsibility?

REFERENCES

Department of Health (DH) (1989) *An Introduction to the Children Act 1989*. London: The Stationery Office.

FURTHER READING

Clarke E. (1993) The Children Act 1989: implications for midwifery. *British Journal of Midwifery*, 1(1):26–30.

Gibson C. (2000) *The Children Act Explained*. London: The Stationery Office.

Miller S. (2002) Child abuse and domestic violence. *British Journal of Midwifery*, 10(9):565–568.

Price S, Baird K. (2003) Tackling domestic violence: an audit of professional practice. *The Practising Midwife*, 6(3):15–18.

Scott L. (2002) Child protection: the role of communication. *Nursing Times*, 98(18):34–36.

Scottish Office (1995) *Scotland's Children: A Brief Guide to the Children (Scotland) Act 1995*. Edinburgh: The Stationery Office.

Simpson D. (1999) The midwife's role in child protection. Part 1: The legal framework. *The Practising Midwife*, 2(3):28–31.
Stower S. (2000) The principles and practice of child protection. *Nursing Standard*, 14(17):48–55.

Finally

THE RIGHTS OF CHILDREN AS LAID DOWN BY THE UN CONVENTION

Legislation and practice in child protection are underpinned by principles derived from Articles of the United Nations Convention on the Rights of the Child, ratified by the UK Government in 1991.

These principles are:

- Each child has a right to be treated as an individual.
- Each child who can form a view on matters affecting him or her has the right to express those views if he or she so wishes;
- Parents should normally be responsible for the upbringing of their children and should share that responsibility.
- Each child has the right to protection from all forms of abuse, neglect or exploitation.
- So far as is consistent with safeguarding and promoting the child's welfare, public authorities should promote the upbringing of children by their families.
- Any intervention by a public authority in the life of a child must be properly justified and should be supported by services from all relevant agencies working in collaboration.

Always bear in mind – Everyone has a duty and a responsibility to do their very best to keep children safe from harm.

Appendix: Useful contacts

Association for Postnatal Illness
145 Dawes Road
Fulham
London
SW6 7EB

Tel: 020 7386 0868
Fax: 020 7386 8885
E-mail: info@apni.org
Website: www.apni.org

Childline
Childline
Freepost 1111
London
N1 0BR

Tel: 0800 1111
Textphone (for deaf children or for those who find using a telephone difficult): 0800 400 222

Childline is a free 24-hour helpline for children and young people in the UK. Children and young people can call about any problem at any time, day or night.

Childline Scotland
18 Albion Street
Glasgow
G1 1LH

Tel: 0141 552 1123

Children's Legal Centre
University of Essex
Wivenhoe Park
Colchester
Essex
CO4 3SQ

Advice line: 01206 873820
Administration/Publications: 01206 872466
Fax: 01206 874026
E-mail: clc@essex.ac.uk
Website: www.childrenslegalcentre.com

The Children's Legal Centre is a unique independent charity concerned with law and policy affecting children and young people. The centre is funded by grants from central government and is staffed by lawyers and professionals with experience in child law. They offer advice and they also produce an excellent series of leaflets for parents and carers caught up in child protection procedures, which are easy to understand.

Family Rights Group
Advice line: 020 7249 0008 (Mon.–Fri. 1.30–3.30 p.m.)

The Family Rights Group (FRG) is a charity set up in 1974 to provide advice and support for families whose children are involved with social services. The group works to improve the services received by these families.

Gingerbread
7 Sovereign Court
London
E1W 3HW

Tel: 020 7488 9300
Advice line: 0800 018 4318 (Mon.–Fri. 9 a.m.–5 p.m.)
E-mail: office@gingerbread.org.uk
Website: www.gingerbread.org.uk

Gingerbread was started in 1970 as a registered charity and is the leading support organisation for lone parent families in England and Wales.

Home-Start
2 Salisbury Road
Leicester
LE1 7QR

Tel: 0116 233 9955
Fax: 0116 233 0232
Freephone: 0800 068 6368
E-mail: info@home-start.org.uk
Website: www.home-start-int.org.uk

Home-Start is a charity, which provides volunteers to visit families regularly, in their own homes, usually once a week for between 2 and 4 hours. They offer a listening ear and offer practical help such as playing with the children or helping the family go shopping.

Keepers of Child Protection Registers in Scotland
Social Work Services Group (SWSG)
Children's Services Division
James Craig Walk
Edinburgh
EH1 3BA

Tel: 0131 244 5486

National Domestic Violence Helpline
PO Box 391
Bristol
BS99 7WS

Tel: 0117 944 4411 (administration)/0117 924 1703 (training)
Helpline: 0845 023 468
E-mail: web@womensaid.org.uk

National Society for the Prevention of Cruelty to Children (NSPCC)
3 Gilmour Close
Beaumont Leys
Leicester
LE4 1EZ

Tel: 0116 234 7200
Helpline: 0808 800 5000

NCH
85 Highbury Park
London
N5 1UD

Tel: 020 7704 7000
Fax: 020 7226 2537

NCH is a long-established leading children's charity. They have 480 projects for children and young people and their families across the UK. Their services include more than 100 family support services and projects for children in care and leaving care, treatment centres for children who have been sexually abused and support services for children with disabilities and their families. Most of the projects are run in partnership with statutory agencies.

NCH Scotland
17 Newton Place
Glasgow
G3 7PY

Tel: 0141 332 4041
Fax: 0141 332 7002

NCH Northern Ireland
45 Malone Road
Belfast
BT9 6RX

Tel: 028 9068 7785
Fax: 028 9068 1020

NCH Cymru
St David's Court
68a Cowbridge Road East
Cardiff
CF11 9DN

Tel: 029 2022 2127
Fax: 029 2922 9952

NEWPIN
National Newpin
Sutherland House
35 Sutherland Square
Walworth
London
SE17 3EE

Tel: 020 7358 5900
Fax: 020 7701 2660
E-mail: info@newpin.org.uk

NEWPIN is a voluntary organisation working with families to help break the cycle of destructive family behaviour. They work through a network of centres where parents and their children develop an atmosphere of equality, empathy and respect. Individuals may refer themselves or be referred by social workers, GPs, health visitors, the probation service or the courts.

One Parent Families Scotland
13 Gayfield Square
Edinburgh
EH1 3NX

Tel: 0131 556 3899
E-mail: stephanie-anne.harris@fife.gov.uk

Parenting Education and Support Forum
Unit 431 Highgate Studios
53–79 Highgate Road
London
NW5 1TL

Telephone information service: 020 7284 8389
E-mail: pesf@dial.pipex.com
Website: www.parenting-forum.org.uk

PIPPIN
Derwood
Todds Green
Stevenage
SG1 2JE

Tel: 01582 883 353
Website: www.pippin.org.uk

Parents in Partnership – Parent Infant Network is a national charity whose main aim is to maintain and improve the emotional health of families through one of the most crucial stages in people's lives, namely the birth of a new baby. This is achieved through their range of antenatal educational classes. They focus on families from all backgrounds.

Sure Start
Level 2
Caxton House
Tothill Street
London
SW1H 9NA

Tel: 020 7273 4830
Fax: 020 7273 5182
E-mail: sure.start@dfee.gov.uk
Website: www.surestart.gov.uk

Sure Start is the cornerstone of the government's drive to tackle child poverty and social exclusion. By 2004 there will be 500 Sure Start programmes helping up to 400 000 children living in disadvantaged areas.

Keeper of the Registers of Scotland (for the parental rights and responsibilities agreement)
Books of Council and Session
Meadowbank House
153 London Road
Edinburgh
EH8 7AU

Tel: 0131 659 6111

National Childbirth Trust
Alexandra House
Oldham Terrace
Acton
London
W3 6NH

Tel: 0870 444 8707
E-mail: NCTinfo@nctrust.swinternet.co.uk
Website: www.nctpregnancyandbabycare.com

Royal Scottish Society for Prevention of Cruelty to Children
41 Polwarth Terrace
Edinburgh
EH11 1NU

Tel: 0131 337 8539

Scottish Women's Aid
Norton Park
57 Albion Road
Edinburgh
EH7 5QY

Tel: 0131 475 2372
E-mail: swa@swa–1.demon.co.uk

The Stationery Office
General enquiries:
PO Box 276, London SW8 5DT
Telephone orders/general enquiries: 0870 600 5522
Fax orders: 0870 600 5533

Bookshops:
123 Kingsway, London WC2B 6PQ
Tel: 020 7242 6393
Fax: 020 7242 6412

68–69 Bull Street, Birmingham B4 6AD
Tel: 0121 236 9696
Fax: 0121 236 9699

33 Wine Street, Bristol BS1 2BQ
Tel: 0117 926 4306
Fax: 0117 929 4515

9–21 Princess Street, Manchester M60 8AS
Tel: 0161 834 7201
Fax: 0161 833 0634

71 Lothian Road, Edinburgh EH3 9AZ
Tel: 0870 606 5566
Fax: 0870 606 5588

18–19 High Street, Cardiff CF1 2BZ
Tel: 029 2039 5548
Fax: 029 2038 4347

16 Arthur Street, Belfast BT1 4GD
Tel: 028 9023 8451
Fax: 028 9023 5401

Victim Support Line
Tel: 0845 30 30 900
Mon.–Fri. 9 a.m.–9 p.m., Sat.–Sun. 9 a.m.–5 p.m.

Women's Aid Outreach
Tel: 0800 587 4761 (office hours only)

Index